The Good Night, Sleep Tight
WORKBOOK

For Children with Special Needs

TODDLERS TO TWEENS

Gentle Proven Solutions to Help Your Child with
Exceptional Needs Sleep Well and Wake Up Happy

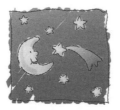

The Sleep Lady®
KIM WEST, LCSW-C
and Katie Holloran, MA, BCBA, GSC

Edited by Maura Rhodes,
former Senior Editor, *Parenting* Magazine

City Point Pr

D1378036

Published by
City Point Press
P.O. Box 2063
Westport, CT 06880
www.citypointpress.com

Visit Kim West, The Sleep Lady, at www.sleeplady.com

Book and cover design by Barbara Aronica-Buck
Cover photo credit: anekoho/Bigstock.com

Paperback ISBN: 978-1-947951-09-9
eBook ISBN: 978-1-947951-10-5

Printed in Canada

First printing

Contents

Introduction

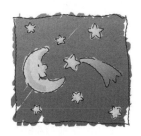 A key factor that makes The Sleep Lady method so successful is that it's not a "one size fits all" approach to sleep coaching. When we work with individual families we consider their values, lifestyles, and child-rearing philosophies to avoid suggesting they do something they would feel uncomfortable doing, and that would therefore likely be counterproductive. We can't stress this enough: A sleep-coaching plan that parents can't stick to is bound to fail.

It's also important to know that The Sleep Lady Shuffle is not an overnight cure. Essentially, you're teaching your child a new skill. So be patient and remember that mastering a skill—whether it's walking, handling a spoon, using the potty, talking, or sleeping through the night—takes time. However, the families I work with solve the majority of their kids' bedtime snafus within a month. (Issues like napping and early rising often take a little longer.)

How to Use this Workbook

For best results, we recommend reading each section of the workbook that's relevant to you and your child before you begin creating your plan (on page 80.) The workbook is organized to first give you the basics of sleep science (Chapter 1), followed by an overview of The

Sleep Lady Shuffle (Chapters 2, 3, and 4). Note that in Chapter 2, where you'll find recommended sleep guidelines for children from the National Sleep Foundation (NSF) and the American Academy of Pediatrics (AAP), you should read the section that matches your child's developmental and cognitive age, rather than his physiological age. If you aren't sure, ask your child's educational or medical team for guidance.

Next, move on to Chapters 5 and 6 to learn tips and strategies that will help you to customize The Sleep Lady Shuffle to fit your child. If you have specific problems around naps, weaning, or co-sleeping, you'll find help in Chapters 7, 8, and 9, respectively. In Chapter 10, you can create your sleep-coaching plan by reading through the examples and then using the template on page 80. Chapters 10 and 11 offer suggestions for implementing your plan cribside and bedside. We've included troubleshooting tips in Chapter 13 to answer some of the questions parents ask most frequently. And finally, in Chapters 14 and 15, you'll find blank charts to use, plus visuals and information about products that you may find helpful.

Now for a few words of encouragement: Your success in sleep coaching will depend on the same factors you bring to parenting every day—consistency, follow-through, and patience—meaning you're as well-equipped as any expert to guide your child with special needs to sleep success. Do be sure that his other caregivers (your spouse, partner, sitters, medical team, and so forth) are as committed as you are.

May you enjoy many peaceful nights of sleep ahead!

—Kim West, LCSW-C, The Sleep Lady

and

Katie Holloran, MA, BCBA, GSC

CHAPTER ONE

Before You Begin Sleep Coaching

Why Sleep Matters

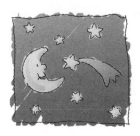

Your child has received a diagnosis from a doctor or clinician and is experiencing problems around sleep in addition to his medical, social, developmental, or emotional needs. It's likely this means he's exhausted, and you and the rest of the household are as well. Perhaps this is your first stop on the way to finding solutions. Or you've already tried strategies to create better sleep for your child that haven't worked. Either way, you've come to the right place. This workbook will provide research-based information, specific guidelines, action steps, and helpful resources to put you, your child, and your family on the path to better sleep.

The body of research around sleep in general, and specifically around sleep for children with special needs, is relatively new, but it's growing. What is known is that parents of children with special needs report a higher rate of sleep problems than do other parents. In one survey of parents of children with a broad range of disabilities, almost 80 percent reported an issue with their child's sleep. Alarmingly, one in four of those parents described the sleep problem as "severe."

Sleep problems, including trouble falling asleep, staying asleep, and getting enough sleep, are especially common in children and teens with developmental disabilities. Between 63 and 80 percent of children with developmental disabilities have issues with sleep, compared to 35 to 50 percent of typically developing young children. Children with

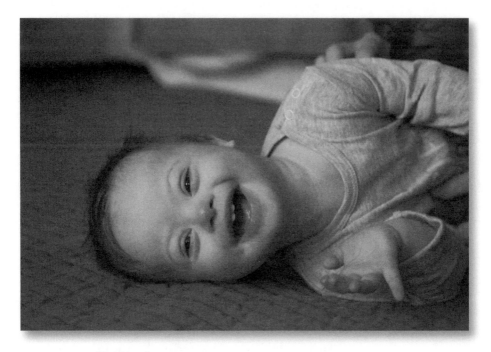

Max, age 2

issues such as attention deficit hyperactivity disorder (ADHD) also struggle with sleep problems more frequently than do other children.

Poor sleep or too little sleep can have serious repercussions for all children, including behaviors such as meltdowns, aggression, self-injury, and repetitive self-stimulatory behavior. Sleep problems also can interfere with learning. Children who are developing normally tend to outgrow their sleep issues, but those with special needs often don't and continue to have associated problems into their teen years and even adulthood, such as obesity, behavioral and emotional problems, and anxiety.

Working with Your Team:
11 Things to Do before Starting Sleep Coaching

1. Rule out underlying medical conditions.

Many sleep problems are behavioral, meaning you can teach your child new sleep behaviors through coaching. However, you should have your pediatrician make sure there are no physical reasons your child is having issues. Reflux, ear infections, and allergies can interfere with quality sleep, for example, as can asthma, which causes the airways to become inflamed and swollen. Even what may be described as mild asthma can take a huge toll on a child's sleep. "If mild asthma has swollen your bronchiole tubes just enough to make you breathe a little faster at baseline, then perhaps your sleeping respiratory rate is 18 breaths per minute rather than the normal 14 to 16 BPM . . . Those extra breaths raise your heart rate, lighten your sleep and fracture your sleep architecture," explains Lewis Kass, MD, a board-certified pediatric pulmonologist and sleep medicine specialist in New York.

Similarly, obstructive sleep apnea (OSA), which in kids often is caused by enlarged tonsils and adenoids (but also neurological disorders, bony problems of the face, jaw, and head, and obesity), can prevent a child from getting a healthy night's sleep by blocking the upper airways. According to Kass, during sleep, this blockage is worse because "our airways and our chest wall muscles and our neck muscles go to sleep too . . . The way a child combats this is to do whatever it takes to open up and enlarge the airway. This is accomplished by waking up in order to take a deeper breath. Accordingly, one of the hallmark symptoms of OSA is restless sleeping."

2. Tweak your child's therapy sessions to make time for sleep training.

Once you've decided to move forward with sleep coaching and have settled on a date to get started, contact each of the therapists and other specialists your child sees regularly. This is important not only because you want to make sure that all aspects of her care complement each other, but also because successful sleep training depends on careful timing, and you may need to reschedule appointments around afternoon naps, say, or switch evening sessions to mornings so they don't happen too close to bedtime. Don't worry about inconveniencing your child's treatment team: Just like you, they want to see your child thrive and are very aware that the better her sleep, the easier it will be for them to give her the help she needs.

3. Review your child's medication.

With his medical team, go over the medicines your child takes regularly to make sure one (or more) of them isn't potentially interfering with his sleep during the day and/or during the night. If this is the case, then the most direct and effective way to address your child's sleep issues may be to change when he takes his medication, or to have him try a different one. Some families talk to their medical professionals about melatonin as well. This is a hormone naturally produced by the body's pineal gland to regulate sleep-wake cycles. While some families have reported success with this as a supplement, make sure to discuss the benefits, risks, and potential side effects with your child's doctor before giving it to him.

4. Keep an activity log.

Because you're exhausted, it's likely your days (and nights) are flying by in a blur, and your short-term memory isn't what it used to be. To find an effective solution to your child's sleep problems, you'll need to get a clear picture of what's happening at bedtime and during the night, what's working, what's not, and how your child is responding. Keep track by writing it all down for a few days or, better yet, a week, before you start coaching. Some parents find it easiest to keep a notebook next to their child's bed. (You'll find a sample log on pages 119–120, but feel free to come up with your own format. Or download

The Sleep Lady's app "Gentle Sleep" for iOS and Android, which will allow you to easily log your child's sleep and also access helpful articles about typical sleep schedules, age-specific tips, and other information.)

Use your log or the app to note when and how often your child wakes up during the night. Include what you did to get her back to sleep, whether you rocked her, nursed her, sang to her, or brought her into your bed. Having such a record to refer to rather than relying on scrambled mental notes in your sleep-deprived brain will give you a more accurate picture of your child's patterns and your own responses, and will allow you to compare your child's daily schedule to the typical schedules outlined in Chapter 2.

Continue the log after you start sleep coaching. Tracking your child's sleep patterns will help you figure out what's working, what's not, and what tactics you should tweak.

5. Determine your child's ideal bedtime.

This is the period of time during which he'll show signs that he's ready to sleep—yawning, rubbing his eyes, twisting his hair, whining. Often parents miss a child's sleep cues, especially in the evening, because it's such a busy time of day. They may be cleaning up the dinner dishes, shuffling through the mail, helping other kids with homework, and so forth. Pay attention to how your child behaves between 6 and 8 p.m. (and make sure he's not zoning out in front of a screen). As soon as he begins acting drowsy, you'll know that that's his natural bedtime and the time at which you should be putting him to bed each evening going forward.

If you have trouble picking up on your child's drowsy signals, you can pinpoint a reasonable bedtime for him by looking at when he normally wakes up and factoring in how much sleep he should be getting based on recommended sleep averages (see pages 8 and 12.) Let's say you have a 2-year-old who tends to wake up by 6 every morning. The average 2-year-old should get 10 to 11 hours of sleep at night, so that means making certain your child has gone through his entire bedtime routine and is *sound asleep* by 8 p.m.

6. Create a relaxing bedtime routine.

Children of all ages need a set of comforting and predictable rituals and routines to help them prepare physically and psychologically for sleep. These activities should be calm, quiet ones, such as reading or being read to, listening to a story, or being sung to. Bedtime is not the time for tickling, wrestling, scary tales, television or other screens, or anything else that's stimulating. Because you're preparing your little one to be separated from you for the night, the tone should be serene and reassuring. With the exception of baths, toileting, and teeth brushing, the bedtime routine should take place in the child's bedroom.

If your child hates some aspect of the bedtime routine, get that part over with first. For instance, if she can't stand brushing her teeth, do it right after her bath, not after you've read two books and she is relaxed and cozy already.

7. Install room-darkening shades.

If your child's bedroom gets too much light, he wakes up very early, or has trouble napping, install room-darkening shades. Leave a dim night-light or closet light on so that you can see him when you check on him.

8. Drown out sleep-disruptive sound.

If your child's room isn't very soundproof and you have a dog that barks a lot, loud neighbors, other children, live on a busy street, etc., consider turning on a white noise machine or a fan, or play white noise or soothing music on your smartphone or other device (there are apps for that). Children do learn to sleep through routine household sounds (and they should to a large extent), but some places are really loud, and some kids are really sensitive. We discourage using music that turns off to mask noise; kids can get too dependent on it, meaning they'll want someone to come in and restart their music every time they wake up.

9. Get your child used to waking up between 6 and 7:30 a.m.

Five days before you start sleep coaching, start waking your child up by 7:30 in the morning at the latest.

10. Get all your child's caregivers on board.

It's vital that your spouse, partner, nanny, and anyone else who regularly takes care of your child understands each aspect of the sleep-coaching plan (and why it's important) and is willing to follow through. This is key to maintaining the consistency that's so vital to sleep success. (See Chapter 7, Nap Coaching, for what to do when you have a reluctant babysitter, and also how to work around your child's schedule if she's in daycare or a school program.)

11. Pick a realistic start date.

Choose a block of time, ideally about three weeks, during which you don't expect any major disruptions or changes in your household, such as trips, moving, or the arrival of a new baby. Some families decide to start sleep coaching during a summer or winter vacation so the grown-ups won't have to juggle sleep training with work. That's a good strategy, but be careful to keep your child's schedule consistent, even if yours is not. For instance, don't introduce a sensible 7:30 p.m. bedtime the very week you plan to let him stay up until 10 p.m. with the grandparents on Christmas Eve, or are going to have a horde of entertaining young cousins camping out in your backyard over the Fourth of July.

CHAPTER TWO

Age-Specific Schedules and Routine

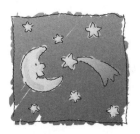

Whatever your child's biological age, because of her special situation she may need to adhere to a sleep schedule that's more appropriate for a younger child. For example, a 2-year-old may do better by following the sleep recommendations for a 12- to 18-month-old. Keep this in mind as you review the following guidelines from the National Sleep Foundation (NSF) and the American Academy of Pediatrics (AAP). They're based on research updated and released by the NSF in 2015 as well as the AAP's 2016 recommendations.

TODDLERS (1 TO 2 YEARS OLD)

General sleep recommendations: Between 11 and 14 hours total, including nap(s) and overnight sleep. Most children take two naps at the earlier end of this age range, then drop the morning nap between 15 and 18 months. Naps at this age should be a total of 2 to 2½ hours.

Some toddlers need a longer transition from dinner to bedtime and should eat earlier than the rest of the family. However, most children this age don't need a meal before bedtime, although some like to nurse briefly (if they're still breastfeeding) for comfort. This is okay, as long as they aren't nursing to sleep.

TYPICAL SCHEDULE (FOR A CHILD WHO GETS UP BETWEEN 7 AND 7:30 A.M.)

7 a.m.–7:30 a.m.	Wake-up and breakfast
9 a.m.–9:30 a.m.	Start of hour-long morning nap (for toddlers who still nap twice a day)
11:30 a.m.–12:30 p.m.	Lunch (depending on morning nap timing)
12:30 p.m.–1:30 p.m.	Start of afternoon nap. About 1½ hours if it's a second nap; between 2 and 2½ hours if it's the only nap of the day
5 p.m.–5:30 p.m.	Dinner
6 p.m.–6:30 p.m.	Start bath/bedtime routine
7 p.m.–8 p.m.	Asleep

CHANGES AND CHALLENGES: DROPPING THE MORNING NAP

Most neurotypical toddlers are ready to give up their morning nap between 15 and 18 months and nearly all children go through a "one nap is too little, two naps are too many" phase. All you can do is make the transition as smooth as possible, although even in the best-case scenario, a child may be cranky and out of sorts for two or three weeks. Your toddler has reached this milestone when she:

- consistently gets 10 to 11 hours of uninterrupted sleep at night. If she falls short of this goal, work on improving nighttime sleep before you tackle the nap change;

- consistently takes longer and longer to fall asleep for her morning nap;

- takes increasingly shorter morning naps or sleeps for too long in the morning and then refuses an afternoon nap.

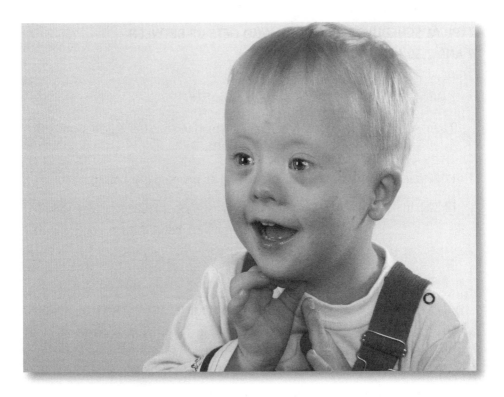

Colin, age 2

Once you see these changes in your child's nap behavior for at least 10 to 14 days straight, you can start the process of dropping her morning nap. It should take only 7 to 10 days. Here's how:

1. Gradually push her morning nap later—until around 11 a.m.— for two days, then 11:30 a.m. for a couple of days, then noon, and so on. Don't let the nap get stuck in late morning. Some kids can adapt more quickly to a noon naptime and others need to go slower. Watch your child. Your goal is for the afternoon nap to start between 12:30 and 1 and to last at least 2¼ to 2½ hours.

2. If your toddler sleeps for only an hour and wakes up tired, then try to soothe and resettle her back to sleep. If all else fails, use one of your emergency techniques, like putting her in the car or stroller.

3. Do not let her sleep past 4 to 4:30 p.m., so as not to disrupt her bedtime.

4. Try to get your child to bed earlier than usual for two weeks or so during the transition—say, 7 p.m.—to cushion her from being overtired.

5. Be open to an occasional "two-nap day." If during the transition your child seems too tired, it's okay to let her nap twice—just limit the morning snooze to 45 minutes.

6. If your child is in childcare or preschool part of the time, try to synchronize the afternoon nap at home with the timetable at school (assuming she starts her nap at school between noon and 1 p.m.).

THE IMPORTANCE OF ROUTINE

A soothing bedtime routine is a must for toddlers. Most kids this age will demand that you do everything in the same order each night, and not leave anything out, so limit the bedtime regimen to a manageable number of elements (one story plus one song plus one cuddle in the rocking chair). Starting around age 2, you may see a lot of stalling and delay tactics. If your child "needs" frequent tucking in, another kiss, etc., respond once. The second time she calls for you, be neutral but firm and say, "No more tuck-ins. Now it's time to go to sleep," and stand your ground: If you say "last time" and then give in, you're sending the message that if your tyke begs and cries long enough, she'll get what she wants. If you and your partner or spouse take turns putting your child to bed, it's perfectly fine if your styles are slightly different. Just make sure that you're consistent about when bedtime takes place and how you respond to delay tactics.

CLIMBING OUT OF THE CRIB

Many toddlers in this age group try escaping from the crib, but it's almost always best to keep a child in her crib until she's at least 2½ and preferably until she's 3. By then she'll have the verbal skills to understand the "big bed" rules and to communicate when she has gotten out of bed for the twentieth time that night. Because children with special needs often reach developmental milestones later than others, note that your own child may benefit from staying in her crib until she's older than 3.

To stop a tot from going overboard (and keep her from getting hurt if she does manage to scramble out), you can:

- Lower the mattress as low as it goes.

- Put pillows on the floor around the crib to cushion falls.

- Remove any large toys or stuffed animals from the crib that she may be able to step up on.

- When your child does get out, return her to the crib with minimal interaction and say, "No climbing."

- Stay nearby at bedtime and peek through the door. If you see your child start to lift her leg, say "No climbing."

- Dress your child in a "sleep sack" so she won't be able to raise her leg over the crib rail.

PRESCHOOLERS (3 TO 5 YEARS OLD)

General sleep recommendations: Between 10 and 13 hours total, including nap(s).

Once your child is in preschool, his schedule will be shaped largely by the hours he's there, when the class has naptime, and other outside factors. That said, there are some things you can (and should) control: Generally, you want him to wake up between 6 a.m. and 8 a.m. (see Chapter 13, Troubleshooting, if your child persistently wakes up before 6 a.m.).

Around age 4, most neurotypical children stop napping. However, you may find that your child needs a nap beyond age 4. Even if your child hits this milestone of no longer needing a nap, make sure he still has some quiet time in the late afternoon (looking at books in his room, for example), and move his bedtime up by about an hour; i.e., if he had been getting to bed at 8:30 at night, now he should be in bed by 7:30. Be open to an occasional short nap when your child seems very tired from a longer, more active day than usual.

By age 5, he can probably stay up a little later—until 8 o'clock—and he should sleep until around 6 or 7 the next morning. In other words, he should get at least 10 hours of uninterrupted sleep each night; adjust your child's exact bed- and wake-up times to coincide with your family schedule and his school start time.

Also, be aware that preschoolers are very good at hiding when they're sleepy, which can make it tough to get their bedtime just right. Continue to watch for sleep cues like yawning, eye rubbing, thumb-sucking, or crankiness. If your tot gets a second wind (meaning you missed his sleep window), start getting him to bed a half-hour or so earlier from now on. Similarly, if he starts nodding off during his bedtime routine or falls asleep the very second you turn out the lights, you're probably putting him to bed too late. Move bedtime earlier by to 30 minutes.

TYPICAL SCHEDULE: CHANGES AND CHALLENGES– DROPPING THE AFTERNOON NAP

6 a.m.–7:30 a.m.	Wake-up and breakfast
	Midmorning snack
12 p.m.–12:30 p.m.	Lunch
1 p.m.–3 p.m.	Nap (if still napping) or quiet time snack
5 p.m.–5:30 p.m.	Dinner
6 p.m.–6:30 p.m.	Start bath
7 p.m.–8:30 p.m.	Bedtime (exact time depending on your child's age and if he still naps)

Some children naturally drop their afternoon nap around the age of 3½ or 4. The main thing to watch as your child gets older is his daytime behavior as well as how long he's sleeping overnight. If your child is sleeping through the night for 10 to 12 hours, seems cheerful during the day, and stays awake in the car or on the bus on the way home from school, chances are he is likely fine without a nap. If you notice that your child is not sleeping through the night, falls asleep in the late afternoon often, and is often frustrated, weepy or extra whiny, try a nap either every day or every other day in order to help fill that sleep tank. Make sure that you leave about 4 hours between the end of the nap and bedtime so he doesn't have trouble falling asleep.

If your child is sleeping through the night and you think he is fine without his nap based on his behavior, it might be time to move away from naps to quiet time. Try to instill about 45 minutes of down-time for your child around the same time every afternoon. Bring books, coloring materials, or quiet toy-play into this routine. You can use a checklist or menu board for your child to use during her quiet time to make choices and play independently. You can try a calming children's video if independent play is hard for your child.

Changes and Challenges: Switching to the Big Bed

Most children move out of the crib between ages 3 and 4. A child is ready to make the switch when he:

- is cognitively at least 2½;

- has mastered the skill of putting himself to sleep at bedtime and getting himself back to sleep when he wakes during the night without any help;

- is climbing out of his crib easily and frequently (refer back to the tips for dealing with a climber on page 12 if you want your tot to stay in his crib longer);

- can say or somehow tell you that he wants a "big boy" bed.

There are different ways to make the transition:

1. The cold turkey approach (removing the crib and replacing it with a bed):

If you do this:

- put the new bed where your child's crib was (if the layout of the room allows for it), *or* place it in a corner of the room so he still feels safely contained;

- install a guardrail on the side of the bed that's not against a wall;

- arrange a few pillows on the floor in case he tumbles out anyway.

A Note about Toddler Beds: Some families use toddler beds (they're sized to fit a crib mattress) as an interim step, but this isn't really necessary. If your child really wants one, fine, but it's certainly not an essential investment. The one advantage is that they're usually too small for a parent to fit in, so you won't have to deal with being begged to lie down with your child.

2. The gradual approach:

- If your crib transitions to a toddler bed, place a stool at the side so he can get out by himself.

- Arrange some extra pillows on the floor for safety.

- If you can fit the new bed and the crib in the same room, you can start with reading books on the bed or have him nap in the bed. Then pick the big night when he sleeps in the bed at night. Once he's sleeping in his bed for naps and nights, you can remove the crib.

3. Some other things to keep in mind, no matter how you decide to make the transition:

- Consider putting a gate on the bedroom door, at least at the beginning, as both a training device and a safety measure. The gate creates boundaries that will make it easier for a child to understand that he has to stay in his bed. It also will prevent him from wandering around and possibly getting hurt in a dark house in the middle of the night.

- Make sure the room is child-proofed now that he can get out of bed unsupervised.

- Let him pick out new sheets or a quilt (or at least give him a choice between two or three sets that meet your aesthetic requirements!).

- Explain the privileges but also review the rules. Make sure he understands that you will still put him to bed, but then he's expected to stay there.

- Be consistent from day one. If your tot gets out of bed, take him right back without any fuss.

- Reward him in the morning for staying in bed: Give him lots of stickers and let him call his grandparents to brag about the new bed.

If you're about to embark on The Sleep Lady Shuffle or some other major nighttime changes, like taking away a bottle or pacifier, consider that it may be easier if he stayed in the crib a little longer. It keeps him in a safe and familiar environment while you're changing other aspects of his sleep, and it may be simpler if you don't have to worry about him getting up and out of bed while you're trying to teach him how to sleep in it.

SCHOOL-AGED CHILDREN (6 TO 13 YEARS OLD)

General sleep recommendations: Between 9 and 11 hours of sleep at night, usually without a daytime nap. The American Academy of Pediatrics recommends nine to 10 hours of total sleep for 6- to 12-year-olds.

Children on the younger side of this range (6- to 9-year-olds) usually need closer to the 11-hour average, and as kids progress through the 10- to 13-year range, they may start needing less sleep, but always at least nine hours.

While it is important to note these averages and arrange schedules and lives to correspond with them, it is also imperative to *watch your child*. Some children may need less sleep, and some may need more. You will know that your child needs more sleep when you see her nodding off while watching TV or when she's in the backseat of the car during afternoon errands. When a kid begins to take longer than an hour to get to sleep it probably means she needs less sleep, but do make sure there aren't any behavioral or medical problems preventing her from falling asleep.

SLEEP-TIGHT TIP

 If you have a new child on the way and you'll need the crib before you think your preschooler will be ready to give it up (even though he meets all the criteria that make it safe for him to do so), make the transition at least two months before the new sibling is due or four months after the baby arrives. If your older child still isn't ready to give up his crib, borrow one or buy a (safe) used one.

Typical Schedule:

6 a.m–8 a.m.	Wake-up and breakfast
	Midmorning snack
12 p.m.–12:30 p.m.	Lunch
3 p.m.–3:30 p.m.	Snack
5 p.m.–5:30 p.m.	Dinner
6 p.m.–6:30 p.m.	Bath or shower
7 p.m.–9 p.m.	Bedtime (exact time depending on age and child's needs)

Be sure to reference Chapters 5 and 6 for additional resources on how to help your child with the bedtime routines, and how to troubleshoot when things are difficult. It's important also to note that you may need to schedule additional time during the bedtime routine for your child to wind down at this age. With school, additional therapies, and activities, our children's days can be extremely busy. Make sure to schedule the time in for your child to effectively calm her body and mind down to be ready for sleep.

CHAPTER THREE

The Sleep Lady Shuffle for a Child in a Crib

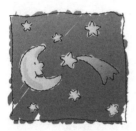

A central aspect of sleep coaching is The Sleep Lady Shuffle. Think of it as a kind of weaning for sleep: You're weaning your child off of what we call sleep crutches, like needing to be nursed, rocked, or held to sleep. Instead of these sleep crutches, you can use the Shuffle to establish more independent sleep practices, without resorting to techniques that may be hard for you to stomach (like letting your child "cry it out"), or that don't fit in with your lifestyle (such as bringing your child into your bed). The main factor behind why the Shuffle works is that you can focus on removing your child's sleep crutch(es), teach her new self-soothing skills, and support her along the way.

The Shuffle can work for kids of all ages. This chapter will be focused on a child who is in a crib, and the following chapter will be focused on a child in a bed.

This chapter outlines The Sleep Lady Shuffle in its standard form. In Chapters 5 and 6, you'll find other strategies to add to the standard Shuffle that will help your child, and Chapters 10 to 12 will walk you through how to create your unique plan using any modifications you choose.

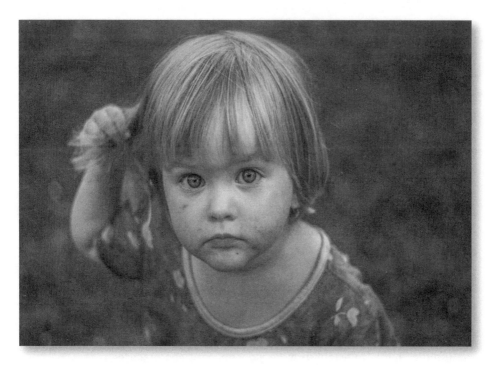

Heather, age 2½

For a child in a crib, here's how it works:

- Start at bedtime, after a good day of napping any way you can get them to, even if that means using the sleep crutches you are trying to change. Go through a calming bedtime routine—nursing or bottle-feeding, a song, etc.—in your child's room with a light on.

- Turn off the lights (a dim night-light is okay) and place your child in her crib, drowsy but awake. For many children this may be the first time they're put down awake enough to be aware of what's happening. If this is the case with your little one, be prepared for tears.

- For the first three nights, position a chair beside the crib where you can sit and easily comfort and reassure your child (see "Guidelines for Sitting by the Crib," on the next page).

Guidelines for Sitting by the Crib

1. **Don't try to make your child lie down (if she's old enough to stand).** You won't win! Pat the mattress and encourage her to lie down. When she does you can touch her and say soothing things like "Sh, sh," "Night-night," "It's okay," and so forth.

2. **You can stroke, sh-sh, pat, rub, etc. your child *intermittently* through the rails of the crib**—but not constantly—until she falls asleep. She'll expect the same treatment when she wakes up in the middle of the night. Take your hand away when you notice your child starting to fall asleep.

3. ***You* must control the touch.** In other words, don't let your child fall asleep holding your finger or hand, because when you move she'll wake up and you'll have to start all over. Pat or stroke a different part of her body.

4. **It's okay to pick up your child if she becomes hysterical.** Stay in her room and hold her until she settles down. Be careful that you don't hold your child for so long that she falls asleep in your arms. Once she's calm, give her a kiss, put her back in her crib, and sit down in the chair. One note: If you pick up your child and she immediately quiets down, then you've been "had." Instead of you training her to sleep, she's trained you to pick her up. Next time, wait a bit longer. You'll know within a night or two whether picking her up helps or further stimulates her.

5. **Stay beside her crib until she's sound asleep at bedtime, and during all night awakenings during the first three days of the Shuffle.** If you rush out of the room the minute your child closes her eyes, chances are she'll wake up and you'll have to start over.

6. **Return to your Shuffle position and follow these rules each time your child wakes during the first three nights** (as long as you and your pediatrician have decided to end night feeding). Go to the crib, give her a kiss, quietly and neutrally encourage her to lie down if necessary, and sit in the chair. Do this at each awakening until 6 a.m.

- Every three days you will move the chair farther from your child's crib (see "Recommended Chair Positions," below).

- During the Shuffle, when you're no longer by your child's bedside but are sitting by the door, for example, and your child wakes at midnight, go over to her crib, reassure her, give her a kiss, encourage her to lie down (if she's standing), and return to your chair by the door. You may go back to the crib to pick her up if she becomes hysterical, but hold her only until she's calm, then put her down in the crib and return to your chair.

Recommended Chair Positions

Position 1   Beside the crib.

Position 2   Halfway between the crib and the door (if the room is very small or the crib is close to the door, go ahead to Position 3 by the door).

Position 3   Beside the door inside the room.

Position 4   In the hallway, where your child can still see you.

Position 5   In the hallway, out of your child's view but where she can still hear you.

Within a few weeks, you'll be able to put your child down to sleep, say, "Good night," and leave the room knowing that she'll happily and easily get herself to sleep without needing your help.

LOVEYS, SECURITY BLANKETS, AND OTHER TRANSITIONAL OBJECTS

If your baby doesn't already have a transitional object—so called because it serves as something familiar to hang on to while switching

When—and How—to Slow Things Down

Children of all ages and developmental stages learn at their own pace, and those with special needs are no exception. So, if you find that after three days of any stage of the Shuffle your child is taking longer than seems necessary to fall asleep, or you sense that she's not ready for you to move your position farther from her crib or bed, then go with that: Give yourself one or two extra nights in that spot—but no more. We generally don't recommend extending the amount of time a parent or caregiver stays in one position by more than two nights to avoid creating a new crutch to replace an old one. For instance, you don't want a child to trade needing you to climb into bed with her for needing you to sit beside her bed in order to go to sleep. The bottom line: It's important to find a balance between consistent movement and getting stuck in one place.

from dependence to independence, according to the AAP—it can be a good idea to help her find one when starting the Shuffle. It's one way to help a baby feel safe and secure while she learns to go to sleep on her own.

Although children often are attracted to soft, huggable items such as blankets (think Linus of the *Peanuts* comic strip) or stuffed animals, what you offer your child should match her sensory needs and preferences. Note what sorts of things your child gravitates toward when she's playing during the day to come up with an item she might find comforting. If she likes smooth textures, you can give her a teether or a smooth-edged toy, for instance. Or if she likes to touch or twirl hair, give her a furry soft toy or a blanket with fringe.

If your child isn't interested in the lovey at first, keep trying to make a connection. Give it a name and a personality and carry it around with you. If she does connect, purchase an identical one in case the original gets lost, and wash the original one often to keep its scent neutral. Or at least alternate the two items so that both smell the same in case one goes missing.

A Note about Multiple Caregivers during Sleep Training:

It's fine for parents to establish different bedtime routines (maybe one isn't into singing but the other is a pro at lullabies, for example). Even so, the bedtime routines of a child's regular caregivers (including sitters, nannies, and family members) should be similar. But while you're sleep coaching, it's generally a good idea for one parent to be in charge of each night waking. If, for example, you're on day five of The Sleep Lady Shuffle, and Dad is sitting in a chair halfway across the room, Mom shouldn't switch places with him after 10 minutes. This can stimulate and confuse the child. That said, it's not necessary to have one person "on duty" all night for middle-of-the-night awakenings. Some couples split the night up or trade off because of their own sleep needs and body rhythms, one taking, say, midnight to 3 a.m. and the other taking 3 a.m. to 6 a.m. One exception: If parent A is tempted to pick up a child who's been crying for 45 minutes after the first wake-up because he or she knows it will put a stop to the crying and allow everyone to finally get some rest, then parent B should definitely take over. Even if this disrupts the process, *a switch is better than inconsistency* or relying on a sleep crutch you're trying to eliminate.

Making the Shuffle Easier for You

Sleep coaching can be overwhelming for any parents, but it's often especially daunting for those who have children with special medical, behavioral, neurological, or developmental needs. Because it's such a gentle and gradual process, the Shuffle tends to generate fewer tears than other sleep training methods.

Even so, your child may protest by crying, which may be unsettling for you. You may be unsure if she is crying because she's frustrated with what's going on or because she's sick, in pain, or something else is bothering her. One way to make the process easier for you is to break it up into mini goals: Commit to only three to five days of the Shuffle. If after that time you see progress, sign on for another three to five days and so on.

CHAPTER FOUR

The Sleep Lady Shuffle for a Child in a Bed

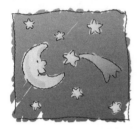 Sleep coaching or doing the Shuffle with an older child who no longer sleeps in a crib can be challenging because there's nothing to prevent the child from climbing out of bed and coming out of their room. Before you begin, here are some things to keep in mind:

1. Don't get into a power struggle. If your child sits up in bed, ignore it; if he gets out, stay put in your chair, pat the mattress, and encourage him to get back in. Do not chase him down or try to physically put him in bed. The door of the room should be shut so he won't be able to wander far. If he lies down on the floor, ignore it. Once he conks out, you can transfer him into his bed while asleep.

2. It's okay to stroke, pat, or touch your child intermittently. The key word here is "intermittently." If you're constantly rubbing his back or stroking his forehead, you can create a new sleep crutch you'll have to overcome. Hands off as soon as you see that he's starting to fall asleep.

3. You control the touch. Don't let him fall asleep while grasping your finger or hand because as soon as you move away he's likely to wake up and you'll have to start the Shuffle all over again. If he reaches for you, pat or stroke a different part of his

body, such as the top of his hand. If he keeps trying to touch you, scoot your body out of reach. You can still lean in to touch or reassure him.

4. If your child becomes very upset, hug him in his bed to calm him, but don't lie down with him or allow him to fall asleep in your arms. Hysteria is not common at the beginning of sleep coaching; the toughest nights will probably occur later in the Shuffle when you're sitting in the hallway.

5. Return to your Shuffle position and follow these rules each time your child awakens at night. Go to his bed, give him a kiss, encourage him to lie down if necessary, and sit in the chair. Do this at each awakening until 6 a.m. Remind your child of his wake-up light or clock if you are using these.

Armed with these tips, here's how to get started:

1. Begin at bedtime on an evening after your child has gotten a nap in if he is still napping. Go through a calming bedtime routine in his room with a light on.

2. After your soothing bedtime routine, turn off the lights (leaving on a dim night-light is okay).

3. For the first three nights, position a chair beside the bed where you can sit and easily comfort and reassure your child (see "Guidelines for Sitting by the Crib").

4. Offer a transitional object (see page 22).

Shuffle positions (you can choose to spend three nights in each position as outlined in the standard Shuffle, or take an extra night or two in each position. See page 23, "When—and How—to Slow Things Down"):

Recommended Shuffle Positions:

Position 1   Beside the bed.

Position 2   Beside the door inside the room.

Position 3   In the hallway, where your child can still see you.

Position 4   In the hallway, out of your child's view but where he can still hear you.

By now your child is probably falling asleep and staying asleep on his own. Your last step is to give him a chance to do this without having you in his room. It may seem like a huge leap, but it's not so big for your child. After all, he's had nearly two weeks of preparation! Move farther down the hall, so that you're out of view but your child can hear you. You can keep making "sh-sh" sounds—not constantly but often enough to let him know that you're close by and responsive. If he cries, check on him from the door. Although it's tempting, don't go over to him if you don't absolutely have to. Be calm and reassuring. Make comforting, encouraging sounds to convey that you're not far away and that you know he can put himself to sleep. Your child really can soothe himself to sleep, but only if you give him the opportunity. You can move to job checks after this. Tell your child that you are going to visit the bathroom, have a cup of tea, or do some other task and that you will be back to check on him later. And then do return, particularly if he is awake and doesn't settle. You can then go back to doing what you were doing, or go back to bed if it is the early hours of the morning!

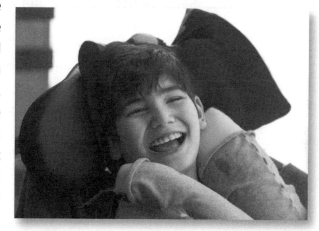

Aiden, age 8

CHAPTER FIVE

Supplemental Strategies to Use with the Shuffle

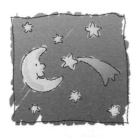 While many families with kids with special needs find that shifting schedules and following The Sleep Lady Shuffle works wonders to alleviate the problems children face falling asleep, staying asleep, or waking too early, others may find they need more. Perhaps their children are drifting off beautifully with the schedule change and addition of the Shuffle, but they are still waking up many times at night, or are wide awake at 4 a.m. instead of sometime after 6. Or, maybe their children are now snoozing through the night, but it takes them an hour or more to fall asleep.

If you find yourself in either of these camps once you've started to implement the Shuffle, try the strategies offered in this chapter to help you overcome some typical roadblocks.

Sensory Activities for Relaxation

For many children, activities that stimulate the senses before bedtime can be physically and mentally calming and help to smooth the way to more successful sleep. A relaxed body and brain can fall asleep faster, sleep longer and more soundly, and benefit from more restorative rest.

It can be especially tough for a child with a challenging physical, mental, or developmental need to settle down enough to nod off and then stay asleep. If this is the case with your child, one (or more) of these activities might help. Try any that resonate with you.

If your child does not respond positively (she gets upset during the activity, you don't see any positive changes in her sleep patterns after a few weeks, or things get worse), don't push it. These are meant to be potentially useful suggestions—not requirements for sleep success.

If your child is being treated by an occupational therapist for sensory needs, ask the therapist to suggest things you can do to help her slow down before bedtime. For example, here's an activity that uses firm touch. It's adapted from *The Out of Sync Child Has Fun* by Carol Kranowitz, who writes that the "children with over-responsivity are often fine with deep pressure and may seek it out. Because it is so relaxing and calming, this is a great activity to do right before and/or just after a more stimulating tactile experience." It's called the Hot Dog, but you can base it on any multi-ingredient food you like—tacos, burritos, sandwiches.

What you'll Need

Sleeping bag, foam mat, or flexible gym mat

Large beach ball or therapy ball

Household items such as clean washcloths, sponges, pot scrubbers, vegetable brushes, basting brushes, or large paintbrushes, or fabric swatches (optional)

Vibrating massager or wooden foot massager (optional)

1. Spread the mat or sleeping bag on the floor or bed.

2. Have your child lie tummy-side down on the mat with her head off the mat.

3. Tell her, "Let's make sure this hot dog is really packed." Then roll the ball back and forth along the length of your child's body (or use the palms of your hand). Use firm, consistent pressure.

4. Give your child the option to be in control. Ask her things like, "Is that too hard? Do you want me to press harder? You can tell me when to stop."

5. Now layer on the condiments. Say, "Time to make you extra delicious. Here's some ketchup!" Rub your child's arms, legs, and back with your hands or with the washcloth, sponge, or vibrating massager if you're using one. Continue by spreading on mustard and adding onions, relish, etc., moving your hands and stroking your child in the direction her hair grows. Invite her to suggest toppings to add: sauerkraut, pickles, even peanut butter and jelly.

6. Finally roll up your child gently and tightly in the mat. Place one hand on her shoulder and the other on her hip and rock her back and forth for a moment. Then tell her, "There's too much stuff on this hot dog. I'll have to squish some of it out." Press firmly on her arms, legs, and back to get out all the excess condiment.

7. When your child seems she's had enough, let her unroll herself while you hold the edge of the mat.

8. For a kid who seems overwhelmed by this activity, you can try rolling and touching just her feet or have her stand while you wrap the mat or sleeping bag around her.

YOGA

Yoga can be a calming and restful activity for kids with special needs (for all kids, for that matter) by helping them to become more in tune with where their bodies are in space and with the sensations in different areas of their bodies. Even a few minutes of yoga each day can be beneficial, but it's especially helpful as part of the bedtime routine.

While there are many kid-centered yoga books and resources to be found with a simple online search, one that's popular with families we've worked with is *Good Night Yoga* by Miriam Gates. It's written for children who are at least 4, but even using some of the poses on your own, without reading the whole book to your child, could be helpful for children who are chronologically or developmentally younger.

Here are two poses that we love for children before bedtime to increase relaxation and alleviate stress. Join your child as he does them—you'll find yourself feeling calmer and more relaxed too.

Viparita karani (Legs Up the Wall):

1. Lie on your back with your knees bent and toes touching the wall.

2. Walk your feet up the wall until your legs are straight.

3. Allow your arms to relax by your side or on your belly.

4. Close your eyes and take deep breaths in through your nose and out through your mouth.

Savasana (Corpse Pose):

1. Lie on your back with your hands by your side, arms and legs straight, feet and hands relaxed.

2. Take deep breaths in and out. Note: If you're doing a guided meditation or mindfulness session with your child as part of the overall bedtime routine (see below), this is a good time to do it.

Guided and Mindful Meditation

Many children go through stages of being afraid of the dark, worrying about having nightmares, and talking about their fears at length. Kids with special needs may find it especially hard to shut out these feelings when it's time to go to sleep. Guided meditation, in which a narrator describes the elements of a pleasant scene or experience, can be an effective way to help a child replace frightening visions with relaxing, calming ones.

Another helpful strategy is mindful meditation—focusing on one specific thing, such as the breath. There is a growing body of literature showing that mindfulness activities can be enormously helpful for children with anxiety or social needs at home or at school.

Here are some apps designed to help children in guided meditation and other activities geared toward mindfulness. All are available for iOS and Android:

Smiling Mind

Breathing Bubbles

Mindfulness for Children

Headspace

Breathe, Think, Do with Sesame

Daniel Tiger's Grr-ific Feelings

Another resource to help kids manage stress or anxiety is the website GoZen (www.gozen.com). Here you'll find animated videos for kids to watch and learn from, as well as articles to help you and your children with relaxation and mindfulness techniques.

You also can find scripts to print out for leading your child through meditation or a guided imagery exercise through a web or Pinterest search.

VISUAL RESOURCES FOR CALM BREATHING

There's a reason breathing has gotten a lot of attention as a calming technique in recent years: Increasingly, research has shown that certain breathing techniques can have a direct and profound physiological effect on the nervous system, essentially calming and regulating the body. Breathing slowly and mindfully activates the brain to send out hormones that inhibit stress-producing hormones, while at the same time triggering a relaxation response in the body.

It's not always easy to learn how to regulate breathing when you're anxious or when it is time to start winding down. Even adults struggle with the concept, so it's no wonder kids of any age or developmental stage may benefit from extra help. If your child has trouble following verbal cues to breathe more slowly or deliberately, for example, or in through his nose and out through his mouth (or whatever technique you're trying to guide him through), we recommend this resource from *The Zones of Regulation,* created by Leah Kuypers, MA Ed, OTR/L, an occupational therapist, educator, and autism specialist.

Coach your child through these visual strategies for mindful breathing. In time he may start to use them on his own: Don't be surprised to see him outlining a figure 8 or a hexagon on his leg or in the air while lying in bed!

The Six Sides of **Breathing**

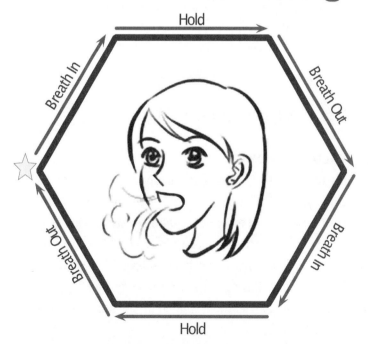

Starting at the yellow star trace with your finger the sides of the hexagon as you take a deep breath in, feeling your shoulders rise as the air fills you. Trace over the next side as you hold your breath for a moment. Slowly breathe out as you trace the third side of the hexagon. Continue tracing around the bottom three sides of the hexagon as you complete another deep breath. Continue The Six Sides of Breathing cycle until you feel calm and relaxed.

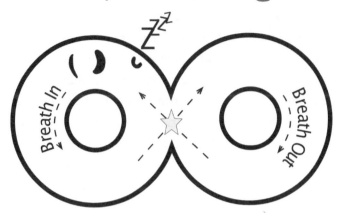

Trace the Lazy 8 with your finger starting at the star and taking a deep breath in.

As you cross over to the other side of the Lazy 8, slowly let your breath out.

Continue breathing around the Lazy 8 until you have a calm body and mind.

Tips to Supplement the Shuffle

"EXCUSE ME" DRILL

This strategy can work well if your child understands what you mean when you say, "I'll be right back," and can then wait until you reappear. It's usually best to introduce the "Excuse Me" drill in the second or third position of the Shuffle, when your child has become used to falling asleep on her own. It will help her learn to relax without you there the entire time. This strategy also can be helpful if you become anxious while sitting in her room waiting for her to fall asleep. Here's how to do it:

After you've gone through your child's bedtime routine and have taken your Shuffle position, wait a minute and say, "Excuse me, I have to go take out the trash/use the bathroom/feed the kitty. I'll be right back." The task you choose doesn't really matter, but it's best to be very specific, so your child understands where you'll be and that you'll be back.

When you begin using this strategy, come back quickly—within a few seconds on the first night. When you do, go to your child immediately, rub her back for a few seconds, and praise her for specific behaviors: staying in bed, acting brave, relaxing her body, etc. Return to your Shuffle position, wait a few minutes, and then leave again after making another excuse. Over several nights, increase the amount of time you're out of the room and decrease the number of times you come back. By not leaving your child alone long enough to become stressed while at the same time increasing the amount of time she's alone, you're gently teaching her how to fall asleep without your being there.

BEDTIME FADING

When it's taking your child more than an hour and a half or so to fall asleep, this strategy can come in handy. It's especially useful for families whose children are older (at least 3—don't try it with a kid who's younger than 2), have limited communication skills, and who do things that are challenging or even unsafe at bedtime.

The first step in implementing bedtime fading is to note on your sleep log how long it takes your child to fall asleep and what time she falls asleep. If it is taking longer than 1 to 1½ hours and she isn't dozing until well after the time you've calculated to be the best for her, bedtime fading may be a helpful strategy. Here are the steps to take:

- Let's say your child's ideal bedtime is 8:30, but she rarely goes to sleep until much, much later. Look back at the past five nights of her sleep log, or keep a fresh record of when she's finally asleep for five nights and use that information to come up with an average time—11:30, for example.

- Make a new (temporary) bedtime for your child that's a half hour later than the time she's typically been going to sleep—in the case of our example, midnight. The idea is to find a time when your child will be so tired that she will fall asleep within 15 minutes without (or with very few) unwanted behaviors.

- A half hour before the new bedtime, begin your child's nightly routine, followed by the Shuffle. Important: In the time leading up to the start of the bedtime routine, engage your child in neutral activities such as reading books, helping with chores, and doing puzzles. Do not turn on the TV or play games that might get her excited.

- Continue this until your child is able to fall asleep within 15 minutes for three consecutive nights. Then you can begin to move her bedtime back toward the ideal bedtime. Do this in 15-minute increments and move your Shuffle position every three to five nights as well.

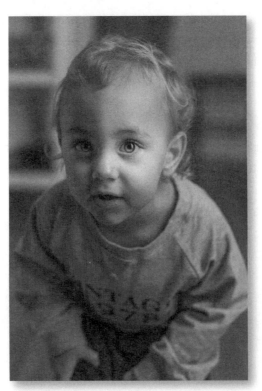

Noah, age 2½

CHAPTER SIX

Visuals for
Bedtime Routines

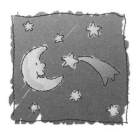

1. Visual schedule or checklist
2. Sleep manners chart
3. Social stories/personalized bedtime story
4. Bedtime passes
5. Visual clock

1. Visual Schedule or Checklist

Visual schedules or checklists can help all children understand what's coming next and how their day will progress. Think about it: If you tell a child it's time to go to the park, she'll probably be very excited—unless it takes 20 minutes to do everything that needs to be done just to get out of the house (pack up snacks and water, go to the bathroom, put sunscreen on in the summer, or coats, mittens, and hats in the winter, get car keys, phones, etc.). By then her excitement likely will have given way to anxiety and misbehavior. But if she knows ahead of time the steps necessary to get ready and leave the house, she'll be better able to tolerate them and feel less anxious.

One way to create a schedule or checklist that will be effective for a child is to include visuals. These could even be photographs of the child herself doing each of the steps in a routine. This type of visual support will be something you will "teach" your child, like any new skill or tool you introduce to her. Get her involved in creating and implementing the chart: what should be included, where to put it in the house (since we're talking about a bedtime routine, posting it near the bedroom or bed makes sense). Go over the pictures with your child to make sure she knows what each one means and do some stress-free run-throughs when it's *not* bedtime.

After a few practices, start teaching the steps on the schedule during actual bedtime. Remind your child to refer to the checklist: Point out which step is first, ask her if she remembers what to do, and offer positive feedback when she responds. If she says she doesn't know or gives a wrong answer, don't make a big deal about it. Use nonverbal cues as much as possible. This could mean simply pausing if your child asks, "What's next?" or pointing to the schedule when she needs help. This will help to build your child's independence so she doesn't rely solely on your voice to do the next step in the bedtime routine. Be consistent: When a visual schedule doesn't work, it's often because caregivers aren't constantly referring to and looking at it. Once you've made using the schedule a habit, your child will too.

Some children need more tangible representations of the tasks that make up their routines—for instance, an actual roll of toilet paper to mean "potty," a bar of soap for "washing hands," a favorite book for "story time." These concrete pieces may help some children understand the routine.

Whether you use visual or tangible representations of the steps of a routine, keep in mind that it will take time and consistency for your child to understand how to follow them, along with a lot of praise—plenty of hugs, high-fives, cheers, tickles, or whatever interactions make your child happy. This will help her to understand that she is on the right track and she'll be ready to do it more often!

Bedtime Checklist

_____'s Checklist

☐	Jammies	☐
☐	Brush Teeth	☐
☐	Potty	☐
☐	Stories+Songs	☐
☐	Kisses	☐

DIRECTIONS: On the left side, check off the item as your child completes it (or have your child check it off). On the right side, paste a picture of your child completing the activity - kids love to see themselves!

You'll find a blank checklist in Chapter 14.

2. Sleep Manners Chart

Most young children love getting rewards for accomplishments. Those with special needs are no exception. If you decide to use rewards as an incentive for your child, tailor them to her cognitive level. Some children are happy to just press stickers onto a piece of paper or wear them on their clothes to show them off. If your child is young either developmentally or chronologically, it will likely be most effective for you to praise him for his efforts to listen to you, follow directions during the bedtime routine, and stay in bed while you sit with him during the Shuffle. Many parents are discouraged by behavior charts when they don't work right away, and often this is because their child cannot understand waiting an entire week for some positive feedback or reward based on their behavior. So, if your child is not able to wait for a reward, consider adding stickers to a piece of paper near his bed every time he shows you he's exhibiting positive behaviors. See if the simple act of putting a tangible sticker onto a blank sheet of paper is motivation enough to keep listening to your directions and staying in bed. Give it a few tries before you decide to give it up.

Some children who are older chronologically or more advanced developmentally will understand and be motivated by a more complex reward system: a chart with squares for each night of a week, for example, to decorate and show off progress. You can keep it super simple and use checkmarks or hand-drawn smiley faces, stickers or stars, and then save a special, extra-big or super-sparkly sticker to celebrate a week of accomplishments.

While some parents do not feel initially comfortable with behavior charts based on past history of them not working, or worries of their children only exhibiting good behaviors in order to get something, many find a chart to organize the goals of the positive behaviors around sleep to be a great tool for themselves, and their children. When everyone in the family can see the behavioral goals that will lead their child to a better night's sleep, it is easier to remind kids about what to do during the bedtime routine and overnight. Whether using a sticker in isolation, or a full-week chart, children benefit from seeing tangible representations of their hard work and efforts to meet their goals.

For sleep coaching, a rewards chart can be an effective way to help a child develop what we call "sleep manners"—desired bedtime behaviors. We call them manners, rather than rules, because "manners" connotes expected behavior and earning praise. Also, it's a reminder that we want to incorporate manners in our life all the time, not just in order to earn stickers.

To create a weekly sleep manners chart, you can simply turn a blank sheet of paper horizontally, write each day of the week along the top (Sunday to Saturday, Monday to Sunday—however makes most sense for your household schedule), and then list four or more manners in a column along the left side of the paper. (See sample below; you'll also find a blank one to tear out and make copies of on page 119.)

___'S SLEEP MANNERS CHART	MONDAY	TUESDAY	WEDNESDAY	THURSDAY	FRIDAY	SATURDAY	SUNDAY
I LISTENED AND FOLLOWED DIRECTIONS AT BEDTIME							
I WENT TO SLEEP WITHOUT MOMMY LYING DOWN WITH ME							
I WENT BACK TO SLEEP ON MY OWN OVERNIGHT							
I STAYED IN BED UNTIL MY LIGHT CAME ON							

Rather than drawings, as shown here, you might illustrate your own child's sleep manners chart with photos of him actually doing the behavior described. Most kids love starring in their own sleep manners chart! Either way, visuals will help him to better understand what's expected and, most important, will limit the amount of talking you need to do during the bedtime routine. Rather than repeating yourself multiple times or risking saying too many words that end up confusing your child, you can simply point or refer them to the chart to know what to do next.

In the beginning, include one easy-to-achieve goal so that your child is guaranteed at least one star and the positive feedback to go with it—such as the "Listen at bedtime" manner in the sample chart. This is a competence builder. It helps your child feel he can live up to the new sleep expectations, that they aren't too hard for him, that *he can do it*. Raise the bar as he improves. Tell him he's so very, very good at getting that sticker that he now has a new manner to focus on.

Review the sleep manners chart every night at bedtime, even if your child doesn't seem interested, and again first thing the next morning. Give lots of hugs and praise along with any stickers he's earned; after a particularly successful night, offer a bonus sticker to wear on his jacket or back of his hand to show to Grandma, the babysitter, preschool teacher, or the bank teller. After a not-so-great night, don't say or do anything to make him feel that he failed. Just say it's okay, he can try again and gently remind him of the behaviors you are looking for and emphasize you know he can do it.

A note about "big" rewards, such as toys or special excursions: Some parents like to promise them if a child earns a certain number of stickers. This often isn't necessary—the stickers, the praise, the hugs, and the sense of accomplishment are plenty. However, if you know that your child needs something more tangible and you would like to have a backup reward, pay attention to your child's cues to see how often to provide this reward. You want your child to feel successful and challenged at the same time. If he's not earning any stars, he may become very frustrated and not see the point of the chart. If you're sure the manners are achievable but he's just taking a bit longer to achieve them, perhaps you can focus on one at a time. Also, look at the Bedtime Passes section later in this chapter to offer additional opportunities for your child to succeed. For instance, if you make one manner "I will go to sleep without Mommy or Daddy," and your child uses fewer than three Bedtime Passes, you can still give a star, sticker, or smiley face in this area.

If you do choose to bring in a backup reward, be sure to make it small, and be realistic. If you promise a trip to Disney World, what are you going to do for a follow-up? You're better off promising a trip to the pizza parlor. You may even want to consider a reward that you could put away if your child "forgets" his manners or regresses. Remind him that he received this reward for having good sleep manners and when he "remembers" them he'll get the reward back.

You can change the manners over time if you need to, but not so often that you confuse your child about his goals. Use positive terms— dos, not don'ts. In other words, say "lie quietly in bed" instead of "don't make noise in bed."

SLEEP-TIGHT TIP

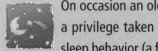 On occasion an older child will respond better to having a privilege taken away as an incentive for changing a sleep behavior (a favorite video, computer time, morning TV). It's a last resort and should only be used with a child who's really resisting making changes or seems not to care. If you have to go there, continue to offer lots of praise for what your child is doing right.

3. [Your child's] Bedtime Story

There is a lot of research showing that a highly effective way to explain routines to children is through narrative formats. Children love stories, especially when those stories pertain to them and even star them as the main character.

In our work, we often use a technique we call "Bedtime Story," which we've adapted from a tool called Social Stories,™ created by Carol Gray, a special education teacher who founded The Gray Center for Social Learning and Understanding. Social Stories explain routines by breaking them down into small steps and explaining those steps in a story format, usually told from the child's perspective using first-person language. We add the child's name into the title to make it extra fun.

To "write" a bedtime story like the one that follows for your child, include details and "plot points" like these:

- Her name, names of other family members, and other personal information: For example: "My name is Brianna and I'm 3 years old. I live in St. Louis, Missouri, with my mommy and my daddy and my kitty, Luna."

- Information about the bedtime routine: "When it's time to get ready for bed, I will look at my nighttime routine schedule":

First, I will take a bath.

Next, I will put on my pajamas.

Next, I will brush my teeth.

Now, I will go potty.

Then I'll climb into my bed with Luna.

Mommy will read us a story.

We will sing our "goodnight" song.

I will give Mommy a kiss and a hug.

She will turn off the lights and turn on the night-light.

• Expectations about the sleep routine and troubleshooting ideas:

When Mommy leaves the room, I will stay in my bed quietly until I fall asleep.

If I have trouble falling asleep, I can cuddle with Luna.

If I wake up at night or before my clock turns green, I will go back to sleep without waking up Mommy or Daddy.

I feel great when I sleep in my bed all night!

When my clock turns green, I will get a star on my Sleep Manners Chart!

Making your child's Bedtime Story a part of the bedtime routine will help her to better understand the routine and what to do when she wakes up or she can't fall asleep at night. But read it together anytime, not just at night.

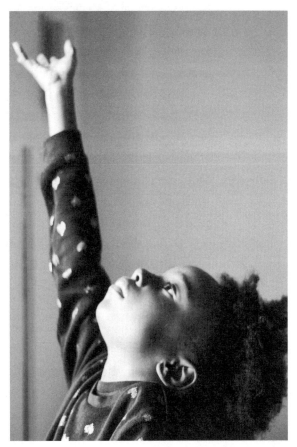

Sam, age 6

To make a story for your child, you can use one of the printable stories from Chapter 14, or download an electronic template on our website (www.sleeplady.com/snwkbk/). The Social Story Creator & Library app can also be downloaded on iTunes for iOS devices. Or you can print out pictures of your child going through the motions of the routine and make your own book. Be creative and make something your child will love!

4. Bedtime Pass

The Bedtime Pass was developed and researched by Dr. Patrick Friman, PhD, clinical professor of pediatrics at the University of Nebraska School of Medicine, and author of many articles and books for parents. While the Bedtime Pass was originally noted to be helpful for children with autism spectrum disorder (ASD), this strategy can be beneficial for any child with special needs.

A bedtime pass is a small card (you could use an index card or blank postcard, or something even smaller) labeled "BEDTIME PASS" on one side with a photo or picture on the other. The image could be of your child or of something he really likes—anything to make the card appealing and fun. Children receive bedtime passes at bedtime. You'll find an example in Chapter 14. A quick Pinterest search will also yield some pre-made printable Bedtime Passes.

During the time a child is trying to get to sleep, or during an overnight waking, he can use a Bedtime Pass for a visit with a parent or caregiver, a drink of water, a hug and kiss, or some other bedtime "curtain call."

To decide how many passes to give your child, for a few nights before you begin sleep coaching, count how many times he tends to get up, asks for water or another hug, or pays you middle-of-the-night visits before settling to sleep. If it's three or more times a night, start with three or four passes per night. Once you start sleep coaching, explain that after he uses all of his passes there won't be any more water, hugs, etc. Then stick to your guns.

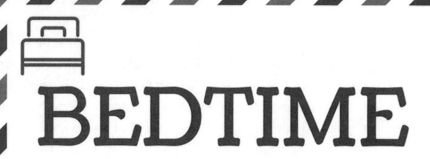

If your child uses all his passes but calls out for one more hug/kiss/drink of water, ignore the request. As added incentive, tell your child if he gets through an entire night without using any passes, he can trade them in for a small reward (a sticker, special dessert, or some such). Decrease the number of Bedtime Passes your child gets each night. Continue to move from many prizes to only a few, and then to just one, as your child learns to put himself to sleep and you fade your presence away utilizing the Shuffle.

5. Visual Clocks/Lights/Wake-up Music

We strongly encourage you to use a toddler clock, a "wake-up clock," or a light with an attached appliance timer to signal your child when it's okay to get up in the morning or after naps. Set the wake-up time on the clock or use an MP3 player with an alarm clock and set it to play a calming song at your child's average wake-up time. Let your child choose the song or consider the "Good Morning!" song from the

Sleep Lady's lullaby CD, *The Sweetest Dreams*, which was written just for this purpose.

Set the clock for 6 a.m. at the earliest and 7:30 a.m. at the latest. **Do not set the alarm for 7:30 a.m. if your child tends to wake at 6 a.m. or earlier.** Explain to her that having this clock in her room is very special and grown-up and she's not to touch it. Show her what it sounds like when it goes off and explain that the clock will tell her when it's okay to get out of bed and start the day. Bonus for you: Your child will no longer spend mornings asking, "Is it time to get up yet? Is it time to get up yet?" If you set it for 6 a.m. and your child starts to sleep through it, then set the time later and enjoy the extra sleep time yourself!

If you don't like the idea of the music or a toddler clock, you can purchase an appliance timer (digital ones tend to be more accurate) and attach it to a light in your child's room. Explain to her that the light will turn on when it's time to get up. Sometimes this is a more effective strategy for younger children and those with less developed verbal skills. And in Chapter 15 you'll find some examples of another option, a Visual Clock.

CHAPTER SEVEN

Naptime Coaching

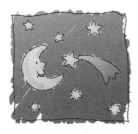 Most children who are 2 and older are only taking one nap each day. If your child is still taking two naps, we will review naptime coaching for two naps here. If you're not sure whether your child should be taking one nap or two, please refer back to the section for toddlers in Chapter 2 titled "Changes and Challenges: Dropping the Morning Nap" on page 9.

It's fine to wait to until after you've done nighttime and overnight sleep coaching before you start the Shuffle at naptime, especially since it can be overwhelming at first. Many families choose to start the Shuffle at bedtime, and then overnight, and save nap coaching for days or even weeks later, once they are feeling more comfortable with the first pieces of the plan. So do whatever it takes to get your child to sleep during the day (take a drive, go for a walk in the stroller, etc.).

However, if you decide to begin nap coaching at the same time you start nighttime sleep coaching, start on day two, or the morning after the first night, of The Sleep Lady Shuffle.

Some things to keep in mind:

- Make sure you're timing your child's naps correctly, based on his age (see Chapter 2). Some families get stuck with timing when a child is taking one nap, and often this nap is around 11 or 11:30 a.m. This timing will be problematic, as your child will then be ready for bed early in the evening, and you will miss his window if you have a bedtime between 7 and 8 p.m. He will be overtired at that point, which will often cause increased or new night awakenings.

- Be aware of your child's sleep cues and windows of wakefulness.

- Do an abbreviated version of his bedtime routine, and include a few calming exercises, especially any that were suggested by your child's occupational therapist (if applicable). Then put your child in his crib or bed drowsy but awake. Sit beside the crib or bed and soothe him just as you would during the night. Try for one hour to get him to sleep.

- Try the nap in the crib or bed twice a day (or once a day if your child takes one nap) before going to a "backup nap plan," which you'll need if you check your sleep log around 2 or 3 p.m. and realize your child hasn't had enough day sleep. You want to make sure he sleeps one way or another for a decent interval before the afternoon is over, so that you're not set up for a bad night. A backup nap can take place in the car, stroller, swing, or carrier, but try to make it different from a habit you've been trying to break. For instance, if you've been working on ending co-sleeping at night, don't put him in your bed for his backup nap. Try a car ride or walk in the stroller instead. Ideally, the backup nap will last at least 45 minutes, and your child will be awake by 4:30 p.m. so that he's ready to sleep at his regular bedtime.

- No naps before 8 a.m.—even if your child has been up since 5! It will throw off the entire day and get him into the habit of getting up too early. This can be a tricky dance and your child may get overtired, but it's worth it in the long run.

- If your child is taking a morning nap, it should last no more than an hour and a half. Wake him if need be, even though it breaks the "never wake a sleeping child" rule.

- Follow the same chair positions for naps as you do at night.

THE THREE MOST COMMON NAP-COACHING SNAFUS AND HOW TO HANDLE THEM

1. **Your child doesn't go to sleep for the entire hour**. Do a dramatic wake-up routine (open the blinds, sing "Good morning!" or "Good afternoon!") and then take your child out of bed. If this happens for the morning nap, he won't be able to last (or wait) until the afternoon for his next nap. Watch his cues: If he starts yawning, dozing while you feed him, etc.—even if it's just 45 minutes after you got him out of his crib—go ahead and try for a nap again.

2. **Your child only sleeps for 45 minutes in the morning (if he is taking two naps)**. This is the bare minimum for a nap. If he wakes up happy and seemingly refreshed, that's okay, but be aware that he might be ready for his afternoon siesta sooner rather than later (after two hours awake rather than three). Watch for drowsy cues so you don't miss his sleep window. In addition, do all you can to make sure the afternoon nap doesn't get cut short. When children wake up happy after a 45-minute morning nap, they often don't wake up happy and refreshed after a 45-minute afternoon nap. If your child wakes up after 45 minutes from his later nap, use the Shuffle techniques to get him back to sleep (try for at least 30 minutes if you can).

3. **Your child naps for less than 45 minutes**. This is a "disaster nap." When a child sleeps for fewer than 45 minutes, he doesn't go through a complete sleep cycle; technically, his wide-eyed state is really a partial arousal, not true wakefulness. So here's the tough message: Go to him and do the Shuffle for an hour—what we call "the longest hour."

Here's an example: You put your child in his crib at 1 p.m., he conks out at 1:30, but only sleeps until 2. You go in and work on getting him back to sleep—which he does, thankfully, by 2:30, after just half an hour. But he only sleeps for 20 minutes. Chances are the negative voice in you is going to say, "I can't believe The Sleep Lady told me to do that! He cried more than he slept. What's the point of that?" But think about it: Your child did it! He put himself back to sleep after a partial arousal from a nap—one of the hardest things to do. Going forward, he'll begin to get back to sleep more quickly and will snooze for longer, if you stick with it.

WHEN YOUR DAYTIME CAREGIVER BALKS AT NAP COACHING

Sometimes nannies, sitters, daycare providers, and even family members aren't comfortable with letting a child cry (even when they're right by the child's side), or don't want to deal with the tedium of spending up to an hour doing the Shuffle after a too-short snooze. If you run up against this kind of resistance, no matter how carefully you've explained the principles of sleep science:

- Ask the caregiver to focus on "filling the sleep tank" as best she can using whatever sleep crutch she's always used before; in other words, have her at least make sure that your child meets the age-appropriate amount of daytime sleep no matter what it takes. If, for example, she generally rocks your child to sleep, then have her continue to do this when putting your child down for naps. Tell her to rock him back to sleep if he wakes before 45 minutes so that he's not having disaster naps all day long. As long as you don't rock him to sleep during the day or night, this can work.

- In the meantime, you should work on nighttime sleep and weekend naps. When you're confident that your child has learned to get himself to sleep, talk to your caregiver again. Explain what your child has accomplished, and ask her to work with you by putting your child down drowsy but awake. If your child is in a daycare center or in preschool, perhaps the provider would be willing to put him down in the sleep area a few minutes before she brings in the rest of the children.

- Note that at some point during your child's overall sleep training, your caregiver's go-to-sleep techniques may stop working. Often, once a child learns to put himself to sleep, the original sleep crutch stops working. Don't panic: This is a good sign— and it also means your sitter will have to join the sleep-coaching team!

And if you or your partner can't deal with nap coaching at the same time you're focused on night sleep coaching, feel free to use backup measures or temporary fixes to get your child some daytime sleep, preferably at predictable times. Nurse him, pat him, swing him, do what you have to do. But don't give up on naps completely or convince yourself that he doesn't need them. As nighttime sleep improves, the daytime sleep might fall into place on its own. It not, take a deep breath and try the coaching again in another month or two, or when your backup measures stop working—whichever comes first.

SOME IMPORTANT THINGS TO KEEP IN MIND

- The morning nap develops first and is easier for a child to achieve than the afternoon nap, so don't miss this opportunity.

- The afternoon nap is more stubborn, so don't get discouraged!

- Look at your sleep log around 2 or 3 p.m. and decide if you will need to go for a backup nap.

- You will be tied to the house during the nap coaching process. If you feel like all you're doing all day is trying to get your child to go to sleep, then you're doing everything right! Hang in there. You can do this!

SOME NOTES FOR NAPPING

If you have a neurotypical child or baby who naps at the same time as your child with special needs, consider implementing *Timed Checks:* Look in on him at regular intervals, basing the timing on your little one's temperament, and be consistent. If you have no idea where to start, try checking on him every seven minutes and slowly increasing the time. When you go to his crib, be reassuring but quick. You'll defeat the purpose if you pat him until he's asleep during your crib-side check.

Go through the abbreviated bedtime routine with your neurotypical child, and then leave the room for a few minutes to check on your child with special needs. You can leave your other child for a bit longer to support your child with special needs during naptime, if needed.

You also may want to consider simply tackling one child's naptime first, and working on the second one after.

If your child with special needs goes to a school or therapy program outside of the house, you may notice he falls asleep in the car on the way home or you receive reports that he conks out on the bus. This often is a sign that it's a good idea to start nap coaching. If your child falls asleep much earlier than his ideal bedtime, try to watch his sleepy cues and respond with a short "cat nap" later in the day or switch to an earlier bedtime. If your child is falling asleep too late on the bus or in the car with you, try to bring in exciting, fun things for your child to do on the way home so that he isn't lulled to sleep in the car.

Here's an example: Your child goes to a therapeutic school program on a bus. He gets picked up at 8 a.m., is put on the bus home at 1 p.m., and arrives at 1:30. During that 30-minute ride, he falls asleep, so he's groggy when he gets off the bus but can't fall back to sleep. You can ask the bus attendants if they're willing to keep him awake during the ride by offering him a snack or playing a game with him. That way you can quickly go through his nap routine when he gets home. If that doesn't work, try for a short "cat nap" around 3, or shift his bedtime to 6 or 6:30 p.m.

If your child is not napping during the week but still seems lethargic on the weekends, he may need a weekend nap on one or both days. This can help your child fill that sleep tank to be ready for the busy week ahead. Having a consistent afternoon quiet time every day that your child is home (between 1 p.m. and 4 p.m.) will help your child nap on days he needs one and recharge with quiet play on other days.

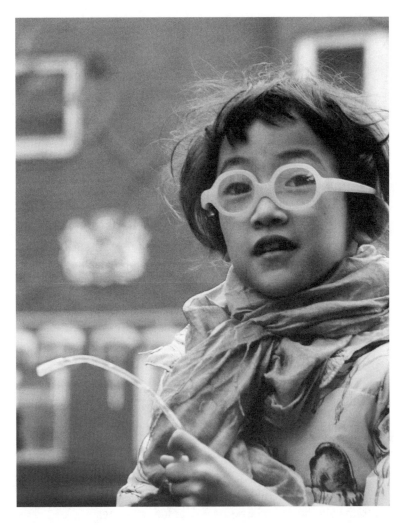

Jade, age 7

CHAPTER EIGHT

How to Eliminate Nighttime Feedings during the Shuffle

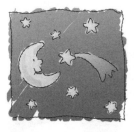 This chapter pertains to children who have an emotional attachment to nursing or a bottle, even though they may not need the calories any longer (meaning they're getting most of their nutrition from solids). While your baby with special needs may no longer breastfeed or drink formula exclusively, she may still be nursing or taking a bottle at certain times during the day, at bedtime, or overnight: It may be the only way she can put herself to sleep, and so it has become a sleep crutch. If that's the case, weaning should be an important part of sleep coaching. Before you commit to the process, though, talk to your child's doctor and other team members.

A NOTE ABOUT FEEDING TUBES

Many children with specific medical needs have feeding tubes during the day and overnight. If yours does, you may not be able to follow the weaning guidance here. Talk to the doctor and medical team about how long your child will be fed overnight. If she does need nutrition during the night via feeding tube, you can work on bedtime with the Shuffle and address overnight feedings later.

Weaning from the Bottle

Take these steps to do it gradually and successfully:

1. **Introduce a cup.** Ideally, you'll have been giving your child sips of milk from a cup since she was between 6 and 9 months old. If not, offer her different kinds until you find one she likes. Some children take to sippy cups right away, others prefer flip-up straws. Others don't care what kind of cup it is as long as it's blue, or green, or has puppies or princesses on it.

2. **Eliminate the bottle, starting with lunch.** Lunch is the meal at which the bottle is probably least important, so this is a good time to serve milk in a now-favorite cup.

3. **Take away the dinner bottle.** Once your child is used to having a cup at lunch (typically after four to seven days), swap out the bottle for a cup at dinner.

4. **Next tackle the morning bottle.** Instead of handing your toddler a bottle as soon as she gets up, go right to the table for breakfast.

5. **Finally, let the bedtime bottle go.** If your child has had a good dinner, she doesn't need extra milk to make it through the night. If she doesn't need the bottle to put herself to sleep then you may be able to skip the bottle at this point, since she's gotten used to doing without it during the day.

6. **When things get rough.** If while weaning your child from the bedtime bottle she begins to protest, take a graduated approach. Begin to reduce the amount of milk in the bedtime bottle by at least two ounces every two days. When you reach the three-ounce mark, offer a cup of water instead of a bottle during her bedtime routine.

You might need to use sleep coaching

This is where you may need to begin sleep coaching at bedtime.

If you're convinced that your toddler or child has to have milk before bed, then work toward serving that milk in a cup and brushing her teeth before she goes to sleep. This will help prevent cavities and fill her belly enough so she doesn't need more to eat or drink from a cup or a bottle. Some toddlers will replace their need for sucking a bedtime bottle with a cup, so be careful!

Eliminate all temptations

Throw away every bottle in the house as soon as your child is weaned. That way there simply isn't one to turn to out of desperation to calm a tantrum or get a baby to go back to sleep at 4 a.m. Don't forget to toss any spares you keep in the diaper bag or car. You don't want your child to discover a forgotten bottle months later and demand a fill-up.

What if your child is just too attached to the bottle?

Let's say your child has developed an emotional attachment to her bottle. Here's how you can tell:

- The bottle is clearly her security object.
- She wants it when she's tired, over-stimulated, or anxious, and she may even whine or throw a tantrum in order to get it.
- She demands a certain beverage in it and a certain amount.
- Your child needs it to fall asleep.
- She carries it around during the day.

To help a child who fits this description break her bottle habit, follow these steps:

- Give her fair warning. Let her know three to five days in advance that it's about time to give up the bottle. Tell her every day, at least twice a day. Pick a time when she's not tired or about to go to sleep. Be calm, caring, confident, and positive.

- Start minimizing bottles. During the period leading up to "D-Day," cut back on the number of bottles she has during the day as well as the amount of liquid in each. Some parents like to restrict the bottle to naptime and bedtime or allow it only in certain rooms. When she's in a bottle "mood," distract her with a game or offer a lovey instead of the bottle.

- Gather the spares. Pick up any bottles you have scattered around the house and stop stockpiling pre-filled bottles in the fridge. Perhaps your child will even help.

- Tell a story. Some parents like to tell stories about giving away the bottles to babies in the hospital, the recycling center, the Easter bunny, etc. That's okay, but you still owe it to your child to tell her in advance.

- Make it official. On the big day, tell your child what you're doing. Remind her that you've been talking about this for several days. Stay firm, and don't waiver—even if she whines or throws a fit—but at the same time be comforting and encouraging.

- Offer a special reward or treat.

- Accept the possibility of backsliding. Don't be surprised if things go well for a few days, and then you hit a rough patch. Gently remind your little one that there aren't any more bottles, and offer a kiss and cuddle, or a lovey instead.

Weaning from Overnight Nursing

Once you and your pediatrician agree your baby no longer needs to be fed during an 11-hour period at night, then choose one of the methods that follow. It should take no longer than a week to eliminate the nighttime meal, so choose a night within that time frame as the one you'll no longer feed her.

METHOD A: THE TAPER-OFF TECHNIQUE

Gradually cut down the amount of time your baby is at the breast. For example, if she usually feeds for 20 minutes, let her go for only 15. Cut back every few nights until she's ready to give it up or until you're down to five minutes: At that point, it's just a tease and it's time to stop altogether. Make sure you unlatch her when she finishes eating heartily, even if it's sooner than the amount of time you've allotted; don't let her just gently suckle and doze. Get her back to bed while she's drowsy but awake.

METHOD B: THE FOUR-NIGHT PHASE-OUT

Whether you're breastfeeding or giving a bottle, feed your baby just once during the night for three nights. It's best to set a rule for when you'll give her that single snack, so you can either:

- feed her the first time she wakes after a set time such as midnight, or

- the first time she wakes as long as it's been *at least four hours* since she last ate, or

- a *dream feed*, in which you wake her for her final feeding right before you go to bed.

Only feed her once at night, and not again until at least 6 a.m., when you can both start your day. If she wakes at other times, sit by her crib and offer physical and verbal reassurance. Follow the "Guidelines for Sitting by the Crib," outlined on page 21.

On the fourth night don't feed her at all. Remember, she's had three nights to get used to receiving fewer calories at night. Usually parents will move their seat away from the crib on the fourth night of the Shuffle, but we're going to modify it for this night weaning. So on the fourth night when she wakes up, sit next to her crib for an additional night. Comfort her from your chair as you did at bedtime. Don't pick her up unless she's hysterical, and then hold her only briefly. If you breastfeed exclusively, it may help to put Dad on night duty: Since he can't breastfeed, your baby might adjust to the no-night-feeding routine more quickly.

Note: Let's say you've decided you'll feed your baby the first time she wakes after midnight. If you find yourself sitting with her and doing the Shuffle from 11 p.m. until midnight while she fusses, don't pick her up and feed her a minute after the clock strikes 12. Wait until she goes back to sleep and then wakes up again—even if she only dozes for half an hour. You don't want to send the message that crying for an hour will yield a feeding.

METHOD C: COLD TURKEY

You can simply stop offering your baby a breast or a bottle when she wakes at night. Go to the side of her crib as outlined in the Shuffle. Just make sure you and your partner are on the same page in this decision. If Mom has been breastfeeding, consider having Dad handle all middle-of-the-night wake-ups, since your child knows that he can't give in and nurse him.

Reducing the number of feedings at night without eliminating them all together:

If you and your child's team think your child still needs to eat at night or you want to reduce nighttime feedings but aren't ready to cut them out altogether, follow the first step of Method B and restrict meals to once a night. Feed your child quickly and avoid other interactions that will encourage her to stay up and play or cling to you.

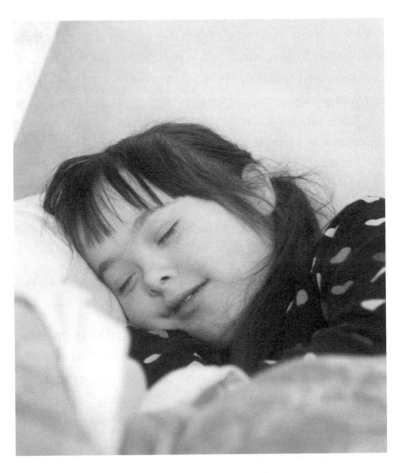

Julia, age 10

CHAPTER NINE

How to End Co-Sleeping

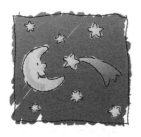

Many families who co-sleep do it *because* their child is unable to put himself to sleep without a parent lying next to him, holding him, or nursing him—not because it's part of their parenting style. It's important to know that it is absolutely okay to continue to safely co-sleep if it's working for you. If your child is sleeping well, and you are too, then don't feel pressured to change this.

However, if co-sleeping is not working for you, you may want to move your little one to a crib or bed in another room. Even if you want to co-sleep, you should still teach your child to soothe himself to sleep. Either way, begin implementing the following strategies at bedtime only. (Don't push it though: If it feels like too dramatic a change, you can work on parts of your sleep plan, such as helping your child soothe himself to sleep while in bed with you.)

We suggest ending co-sleeping in stages. Start by getting your child on board. If he's old enough, prepare him by talking through the imminent change. Even a 1-year-old can comprehend more than you realize, and certainly by 18 months or so kids can understand a good deal. Let your child know what's coming and make it sound enticing and exciting. For an older child, sticker charts and rewards are great incentives.

STAGE ONE: DAYTIME AND PLAYTIME

Get your child used to his room when he is awake and in daylight. In fact, he shouldn't just be used to it, he should like it. Play with him there, change him there, hug him and kiss him there. If the room he'll be sleeping in alone is unfamiliar and he needs incentives to venture there, buy him some fun new toys or check some books out of the library. (You can skip this stage if your child is already playing and/or napping in his room.)

STAGE TWO: NAPPING

If your child is not already napping in his bedroom, start now. Spend a week or two getting him accustomed to napping in his own crib or bed during the day, before you make the nighttime transition. Lie down with him in his room for two or three days if your intuition tells you he needs that extra assistance. If he has trouble falling asleep in his room and you don't want to lie down with him, sit with him for the next few days, but try to be a fairly neutral presence. Calm and soothe him but don't let him constantly engage you, or all the interaction will be an excuse for him not to sleep. After a few days, try The Sleep Lady Shuffle for nap training. If you do, note that it's up to you whether you want to address the napping first, or napping and nighttime sleep simultaneously—it doesn't matter if you are sitting in exactly the same position day and night at this point.

Instead of the Shuffle, you have the option of trying to settle your child for a nap with his lovey, then leaving the room, checking on him every five minutes if he's crying. If that feels abrupt, remember that either approach is fine, and that you should choose the one that feels best for you and suits your child. Read the chapter for your child's age for details on the Shuffle and nap coaching.

STAGE THREE: CO-SLEEPING IN YOUR CHILD'S ROOM

When you and your child are ready for night training—and it will be clear; we're talking days or weeks, not months—you should start The Sleep Lady Shuffle, with one extra preliminary phase: Spend up to three nights sleeping in his room with him to create a bridge between the family bed and independent sleep. Throw a mattress on the floor, drag in the guest bed, and pile up some sleeping bags—whatever is safe and comfortable for both of you to sleep on.

STAGE FOUR: START THE SLEEP LADY SHUFFLE

Once you've gone through your usual bedtime routine, put your child in his bed or crib. Sit next to the crib or bed to soothe him. Pat him or rub his back intermittently, but don't relent and bring him into your bed or into the makeshift bed on the floor. Stay next to his crib or bed until he is completely asleep.

You can sleep in his room on the makeshift bed if that will make you more comfortable and consistent, but only for two or three nights. Any longer, and he'll have an even harder time adjusting when you leave. If your child is in a bed and he gets out and tries to join you on the floor, put him back immediately without a word. If he does this repeatedly or if you wake up at night and find he's in bed with you, skip ahead to the Shuffle step where you sit in a chair; remove the makeshift bed and stop sleeping in his room.

Each time your child wakes during the night, return to his bed to offer physical and verbal reassurance until he goes back to sleep. Sit next to your child's crib or bed for three nights to soothe him. Every three nights move a little farther away so that he can gradually fall asleep more independently. Move across the room, then to the doorway, then out the door into the hall, until finally you're able to leave him alone while still checking on him frequently.

CHAPTER TEN

Creating Your Plan

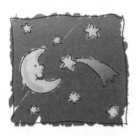 Now it's time to devise your own sleep coaching plan! We encourage parents to create their plan together and during the waking hours. Think it through, talk it through, and write it down. Putting it on paper will keep you both on the same page (literally and figuratively!) and make it less likely you'll have a misunderstanding. Most important, it will help you be consistent with your child.

Following are sample plans—one for a 22-month-old who's still in a crib and another for a 7-year-old who sleeps in a bed.

MEET LINUS, 22 MONTHS OLD, SLEEPING IN A CRIB

Linus has been diagnosed with a developmental delay. He receives home-based therapy during the day with an occupational therapist and a physical therapist to work on fine and gross motor skills. Linus is usually put down in his crib between 8:45 and 9 p.m. after falling asleep with a bottle while being held. He wakes up two to six times per night, and is usually up for the day around 6:30 a.m. When he wakes up at night, his mom or dad sometimes pick him up and try to get him to fall asleep in their arms, or sometimes they prepare a bottle and feed him back to sleep. They also have tried letting him cry, but after 45 minutes they usually are at their wits' end and fall back on giving him a bottle so that everyone can get some rest. Linus no longer has a bottle during the day.

OUR PLAN FOR LINUS

We have met with the following specialists on our child's team:

Occupational therapist, pediatrician, physical therapist.
We have discussed our child's eating, growth, medications, therapies, and general health.

We have ruled out any potential underlying medical conditions that may be interfering with our child's sleep. Our team has consulted with us about any current medical needs, interventions, and medications. We have discussed medications as well as the dosage and timing of them, and have decided to make the following changes, or have been given the green light to move forward.

Linus is not currently taking medications.

We have discussed any possible underlying medical issues, and have been given the green light to move forward from the pediatrician.

After reviewing the sleep averages, we have found that our child requires on average the following amount of sleep:

Total amount of nighttime sleep:	11–11.5 hours
Total amount of daytime sleep:	1.5–2 hours
Number of naps:	1

After reviewing our child's eating and sleep
logs from the last few days, we believe
his natural bedtime window is: 7:30 p.m.

We will be working toward an approximate eating and sleeping schedule as outlined on the next page.

6:30–7 a.m.	Wake-up range
7 a.m.	Breakfast/Feeding
2–3 hours	Window of wakefulness
9 a.m. (1.5– 2 hours)	Morning nap (minimum length–maximum length)
12–12:30 p.m.	Lunch/Feeding
2–3 hours	Window of wakefulness
1:30–2pm (1–1.5 hours)	Afternoon nap (minimum length–maximum length)
4 hours	Window of wakefulness to bedtime
3–3:30 p.m.	Snack
n/a	Optional third nap? timing/duration?
5:30 p.m.	Dinner/Feeding
6:15 p.m.	Start of bedtime routine
7–7:15 p.m.	Lights out in bed

BEDTIME ROUTINE WORKSHEET

Our bedtime routine will include the following (we have added steps based on therapist recommendations, where applicable):

Time Mom home:	**5 p.m.**
Time Dad home:	**5:30 p.m.**
Time Linus needs to be in bed and falling asleep:	**7–7:15 p.m.**

List everything that needs to happen before bed (include any sensory strategies, and allot time for them as well):

1. dinner

2. play/read books

3. bath

4. brush teeth

5. diaper change

6. jammies

7. wash hands

8. read book

9. prayers

10. Hot Dog

11. extra massage, if needed

12. bottle (will switch to cup of milk in a few months)

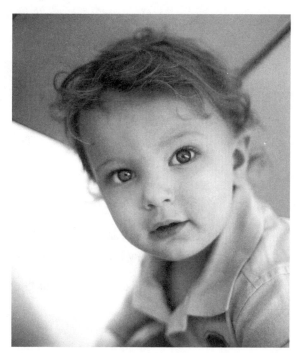

Nicholas, age 2

Use this table to create the evening schedule:

TIME	ACTIVITY	DURATION	LEAD ADULT
5:00 p.m.	Mom arrives home, starts dinner prep	20 minutes	Mom
5:30 p.m.	Dad arrives home + Dinner	20 minutes	Mom and Dad
5:50 p.m.	Play/Read	25 minutes	Mom and Dad
6:15 p.m.	Bath	10 minutes	Mom
6:25 p.m.	Jammies	5 minutes	Dad
6:30 p.m.	Brush teeth	5 minutes	Dad
6:35 p.m.	Diaper change	5 minutes	Dad
6:40 p.m.	Read book + prayers, Bottle	10 minutes	Mom and Dad
6:50 p.m.	Hot Dog and extra massage	10 minutes	Mom and Dad
7:00 p.m.	Lights Out/Shuffle Position		Alternate

If applicable, we have created a sleep manners sticker chart with the following manners and will use the resource in Chapter 14 to print it out prior to starting coaching (limit to 3 or 4 manners maximum): **N/A**

We will add these visuals to the bedtime and/or nighttime routine:

- We will create a Bedtime Story for Linus and read that as part of story time after dinner or pre-bed.

- We will create a Bedtime Checklist for Linus.

OUR BEDTIME PLAN

- We will sit in the Shuffle position and follow the Shuffle rule.

- We will alternate nights leading to bedtime. The person on duty will decide when it is appropriate to pick up Linus to calm him, and will determine if it helps him.

- The off-duty parent will not coach the on-duty parent from the doorway and will support efforts knowing that the other parent loves Linus and is a caring parent to him.

- We will add one extra night to each position, except for by the door, when we will add 2 extra nights:

  - Nights 1–4 by the crib.

  - Nights 5–9 by door (his room is small and his crib is near the door so a halfway position isn't necessary).

  - Nights 10–13 hallway in view. He can see us from his crib.

  - Nights 14–17 hallway out of view with his door open a crack to a few inches.

  - Nights 18 and beyond—leave and shush intermittently from doorway if still necessary.

OUR NIGHTTIME STRATEGY (Will you be feeding your child during the night? If yes, outline the feeding plan and who will be doing it.)

- We will not feed Linus overnight, as feeding to sleep is the crutch, and he does not need to eat overnight. We will do a Set Time Feed at midnight or later, for the first 3 nights. If Linus wakes up during the night before midnight, or after the feeding, Dad will go to the Shuffle position and wait for him to fall asleep. Mom will not coach from the hallway.

OUR NAP PLAN (review Chapter 7, Naptime Coaching):

We will follow the Shuffle for naps.

WE PLAN TO BEGIN NAP COACHING ON:

The day after the night we start coaching.

OUR SHORTENED PRE-NAP ROUTINE WILL BE:

- Book/Bottle
- Hot Dog/Massage

OUR BACKUP NAP PLAN IS:

Car ride

OUR DAYCARE PROVIDER/SCHOOL TEAM HAS AGREED TO OUR PLAN.

Maria, Linus's nanny, will follow the plan and the Shuffle.

OUR THERAPY TEAM HAS AGREED TO (ANY CHANGES IN SCHEDULE OR SUPPORT WITH ROUTINES OR SLEEP STRATEGIES):

We are moving PT from 5:30–6:30 on Wednesday nights to 8–9 a.m. on Saturdays.

OUR DOCTOR WILL BE MONITORING OUR FEEDING AND SLEEP PROGRESS.

We will keep our feeding and sleeping logs, and will bring them to the pediatrician's office for our visits.

MEET LEXI, 7 YEARS OLD, SLEEPS IN A BED

Lexi has been diagnosed with ADHD and is on the autism spectrum. Her parents have been focused on getting her the therapy and educational support she needs and are now ready to help her sleep. Lexi has fallen asleep independently a few times in her life, but usually one of her parents has to lie down with her for her to fall asleep. Mom and Dad have tried to stay out of Lexi's bed overnight, but when she wakes up crying at midnight, 1 a.m., 2 a.m., 3 a.m., they eventually sleep in her bed so everyone can get some rest. Lexi is one of three children, and her parents are truly exhausted.

OUR PLAN FOR LEXI

We have met with the following specialists on our child's team: Pediatrician, speech therapist, occupational therapist, ABA therapist.

We have discussed our child's eating, growth, medications, therapies, and general health.

We have ruled out any potential underlying medical conditions that may be interfering with our child's sleep. Our team has consulted with us about any current medical needs, interventions, and medications. We have discussed medications as well as the dosage and timing of them, and have decided to make the following changes or have been given the green light to move forward.

Lexi is on medication for ADHD. We discussed dosage with the pediatrician. We have agreed to move the timing to the morning instead of the evening, and we will be diligent in logging with eating, sleeping, and other behaviors so we don't negatively affect anything with the timing change.

After reviewing the sleep averages, we have found that our child requires the following amount of sleep:

Total amount of nighttime sleep: **We believe Lexi needs 10½–11 hours of sleep at night.**

Total amount of daytime sleep: **Lexi does not need daytime sleep (although she falls asleep in the car on the way home a lot, which is why we know she needs more sleep at night).**

Number of naps: **0**

After reviewing our child's eating and sleep logs from the last few days we believe his/her natural bedtime window is: **8 p.m.**

We will be working toward an approximate eating and sleeping schedule as outlined on the next page.

6:30–7 a.m.	Wake-up range
7 a.m.	Breakfast/Feeding
All day	Window of wakefulness
n/a	Morning nap (minimum length–maximum length)
12–12:30 p.m.	Lunch/Feeding
All day	Window of wakefulness
n/a	Afternoon nap (minimum length–maximum length)
All day	Window of wakefulness to bedtime
3:30 p.m.	Snack
n/a	Optional third nap? Timing/duration?
5:30 p.m.	Dinner/Feeding
6:45 p.m.	Start of bedtime routine
7:30–7:45 p.m.	Lights out in bed

BEDTIME ROUTINE WORKSHEET

Our bedtime routine will include the following (we have added steps based on therapist recommendations where applicable):

Time Mom home:	**5:30 p.m.**
Time Dad home:	**4 p.m. (with kids)**
Time Lexi needs to be in bed falling asleep:	**7:30 p.m.**

List everything that needs to happen before bed (include any sensory strategies, and allot time for them as well):

1. homework

2. dinner

3. shower

4. brush teeth

5. bathroom/wash hands

6. book

7. songs

8. prayers

9. deep pressure massage

10. swing time

Use this table to create the evening schedule:

TIME	ACTIVITY	DURATION	LEAD ADULT
4:00 p.m.	Dad arrives home with kids; works with Lexi on homework while other kids do homework independently		
		1 hour	Dad
5:00 p.m.	Dinner Prep	30 minutes	Dad
5:30 p.m.	Mom home + Dinner	30 minutes	Mom and Dad
6:00 p.m.	Swing for Lexi, Bedtime routine (baths) for siblings		
		30 minutes	Dad—Lexi Mom—siblings
6:30 p.m.	Siblings reading time, Lexi shower		
		20 minutes	Mom—Lexi Dad—siblings
6:50 p.m.	Lights out–siblings, Lexi jammies		
		10 minutes	Mom—Lexi Dad—siblings
7:00 p.m.	Lexi brush teeth, potty, and wash hands		
		10 minutes	Mom and Dad
7:10 p.m.	Lexi deep pressure massage		
		5 minutes	Mom and Dad
7:15 p.m.	Lexi 2 books, 2 songs, 2 prayers		
		10 minutes	Mom and Dad
7:25 p.m.	Lights out Lexi		Mom and Dad

If applicable, we have created a sleep manners sticker chart with the following manners and will use the resource in Chapter 14 to print it out prior to starting coaching (limit to 3 or 4 maximum):

- I followed directions at bedtime.

- I fell asleep without Mommy or Daddy in bed with me.

- I fell back to sleep without Mommy or Daddy in bed with me.

- I stayed asleep until my wake-up light came on!

We will add these visuals to the bedtime and/or nighttime routine:

Clock	Bedtime Story
Routine Checklists	Bedtime Passes

Our child's current sleep crutch is:

Mom and Dad sleeping in bed with her (either at bedtime or overnight when we're exhausted)

OUR BEDTIME PLAN

- Mom and Dad will have a family meeting and discuss with Lexi the sleep manners that are expected of her. We will also tell her that we will no longer be lying down with her at bedtime or during the night, but that we will stay with her while she learns to put herself to sleep.

- Mom and Dad will alternate nights and will discuss this prior to bedtime.

- On the first night Mom will review Lexi's sleep manners before turning off the lights. Mom will sit by Lexi's bed at bedtime until she falls asleep.

- Once lights are out there will be little engagement or discussions with Lexi. She will be given 2 Bedtime Passes for covering up, bathroom, water, an extra hug, and after that the passes run out.

- Mom and Dad have reviewed all the rules of the Shuffle outlined on pages 25–26.

- Mom will move away from the bedside if Lexi continues to put her legs on her or tries to put her head on her lap and will not be redirected.

- Mom will hug Lexi to calm her down if needed, but will not lie down with her.

- Mom and Dad agree to be a united front and consistent with Lexi, knowing that this will help her.

- We acknowledge that changing sleep habits in a 7-year-old can take longer.

- Mom and Dad agree that learning to put yourself to sleep is an essential life skill and that it is one of our tasks as parents to teach Lexi.

OUR CHAIR POSITIONS WILL BE: We will be spending 5 nights in each position. We will modify the first position to be sitting on Lexi's bed.

- Nights 1–5 sitting on bed.
- Nights 6–10 by the bed.
- Nights 11–15 by door. If Lexi continues to get out of the bed when we are sitting at the door we will stand, count to 3, and say, "Lexi, I will not sit in your room unless you stay in your bed quietly. I will count to 3 and if you are not in your bed I will leave and shut the door." If we have to leave and shut the door we will count to 10 and open the door and tell Lexi, "If you get in your bed I will come and sit in your room." We will say this in a calm but firm voice. We will do this as often as necessary until she gets back into the bed.

- Nights 16–20 hallway in view. She can see us from her bed. We realize this may be the most difficult phase for Lexi. We will respond the same way as outlined above if she gets out of the bed.

- Nights 21–25 hallway out of view, with her door open a crack to a few inches. We will use our voice intermittently to reassure her of our presence if necessary.

- Nights 26 and on—leave and do "job checks." We will tell her that we will check on her after we brush our teeth, for example. We will stay upstairs in our room for a few nights until she is asleep and then progress to going downstairs.

OUR NIGHTTIME STRATEGY IS: (will you be feeding your child during the night? If yes, outline the feeding plan and who will be doing it.)

- Each time Lexi wakes and gets out of her bed we will take her hand and walk her back to her bed.

- Each time she wakes up before 6 a.m. we will tell her calmly that "Your clock light is not on, which means it's still nighttime so you must go back to sleep in your bed."

- We will sit by her bed until she is asleep for the first three nights and follow the above chair positions. We will experiment with Timed Checks as well.

OUR NAP PLAN IS: (review Chapter 7, Naptime Coaching)

We plan to begin nap coaching on: **N/A**

Our shortened pre-nap routine will be: **N/A**

Our backup nap plan is: **N/A**

Our daycare provider/school team has agreed to:

Ask Lexi how she is doing on her Manners Chart, and celebrate her successes.

Our therapy team has agreed to: (any changes in schedule or support with routines or sleep strategies)

All of our therapists will be checking on our progress and celebrating Lexi's success. Right now, therapy timing works with her sleep schedule, but we will continue to monitor with therapy and medications.

Our doctor will be monitoring:

Medication change: We will continue to provide logs and discuss how it's going.

Our Plan for _____
(your child's name here)

We have met with the following specialists on our child's team:

We have discussed our child's eating, growth, medications, therapies, and general health.

We have ruled out any potential underlying medical conditions that may be interfering with our child's sleep. Our team has consulted with us about any current medical needs, interventions, and medications. We have discussed medications as well as the dosage and timing of them, and have decided to make the following changes or have been given the green light to move forward.

After reviewing the sleep averages, we have found that our child requires on average the following amount of sleep:

Total amount of nighttime sleep:

Total amount of daytime sleep:

Number of naps:

After reviewing our child's eating and sleep logs over the last few days we believe his/her natural bedtime window is: _____ p.m.

We will be working toward an approximate eating and sleeping schedule as outlined on the next page.

_____	Wake-up range:
_____	Breakfast/Feeding
_____	Window of wakefulness
_____	Morning nap (minimum length–maximum length)
_____	Lunch/Feeding
_____	Window of wakefulness
_____	Afternoon nap (minimum length–maximum length)
_____	Window of wakefulness to bedtime
_____	Snack
_____	Optional third nap? Timing/duration?
_____	Dinner/Feeding
_____	Start of bedtime routine
_____	Lights out in bed

BEDTIME ROUTINE WORKSHEET

Our bedtime routine will include the following (we have added pieces based on therapist recommendations, where applicable):

Time Mom home:

Time Dad home:

Time _____ needs to be in bed falling asleep:

List everything that needs to happen before bed (include any sensory strategies, and allot time for them as well).

Use this table to create the evening schedule:

TIME	ACTIVITY	DURATION	LEAD ADULT
5pm	Mom arrives home, starts dinner prep	20 minutes	Mom
5:30 pm			
6:00 pm			
6:30 pm			
7:00 pm			
7:30 pm			

If applicable, we have created a sleep manners sticker chart with the following manners and will use the resource in Chapter 14 to print it out prior to starting coaching (limit to 3 or 4 maximum):

1.
2.
3.
4.

We will add these visuals to the bedtime and/or nighttime routine:

1.
2.
3.
4.

Our child's current sleep crutch is:

_____

Our bedtime plan is:

_____

Our chair positions will be:

_____

Our nighttime strategy is: (will you be feeding your child during the night? If yes, outline the feeding plan and who will be doing it.)

_____

Our nap plan is: (review Chapter 7, Naptime Coaching)

_____

We plan to begin nap coaching on:

_____

Our shortened pre-nap routine will be:

1._____
2._____
3._____

Our backup nap plan is:

_____

Our daycare provider/school team has agreed to:

_____

Our therapy team has agreed to: (any changes in schedule or support with routines or sleep strategies)

_____

Our doctor will be monitoring:

_____

We're ready to go! We have blocked out four weeks of our schedule and are dedicating ourselves to improving our child's sleep habits! There is sleep for all at the end of the tunnel!

CHAPTER ELEVEN

Implementing Your Plan for a Child in a Crib

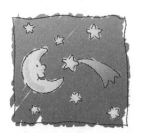

POSITION 1 (NIGHTS ONE THROUGH THREE, FOUR, OR FIVE, DEPENDING ON YOUR PLAN)

Once bath, stories, bottle/nursing, checklist, bedtime story, and songs are over, sit in a chair right **beside your child's crib**. If she cries or fusses, you can touch her. It's important that you control the physical touch; for instance, rather than let your child hold your finger, *you* should pat *her*. Take care not to touch her constantly, though (tempting as it will be!). You don't want to swap one association, like rocking, for another, such as a constant caress or the sound of your voice. Another reason to keep touch to a minimum is that on day four, you'll be moving your chair away from the side of the crib, and frequent contact won't be possible.

Try not to pick her up, but if she becomes extremely upset, hold her by leaning over the side of the crib rather than lifting her out. Keep the cuddle brief: Hold her until she's calm but then put her back down while she's still awake. Limit verbal comforting to soothing shushing, and save singing and lullabies for the bedtime routine. Try closing your own eyes. Doing so may make it easier not to talk to her, and it also conveys the message that it's time to sleep. In other words, be as boring as possible. Stay there until she falls asleep.

When your child wakes up at night during the Shuffle (as she will in the beginning), go to her crib and try to calm her. If she's sitting up or standing, encourage her to lie down. If she doesn't settle, sit in the chair by her crib and stay there until she goes back to sleep. Do this for each waking until 6 a.m. (the earliest), when you can both start your day.

If your child has a particularly rough night, don't stop the sleep training. But you may want to let her take a longer nap or an extra one the next day so she's not overtired for the next night. Provide the extra naptime within the sample timelines outlined in Chapter 2. Let's say your 1-year-old has been up since 5 a.m. On a normal day, she would start her first nap of the day around 9 a.m., but on this day, she'll be too tired to stay awake until 9. Don't force it, let her snooze at 8 a.m. at the earliest—but don't throw her schedule completely out of whack by letting her nap at 6:30 a.m. If she takes a third little nap in late afternoon or naps a half-hour longer than usual, that's fine. Similarly, if your preschooler normally naps from 1 p.m. to 3, it's okay to let her sleep until 4 p.m. if she needs it after a hard night or a too-early morning—but don't let her snooze all the way until dinner or nap before noon.

Another way of handling a temporary sleep deficit is to put your child to bed a little earlier than usual for a few nights. In short, watch her, trust yourself, and make some commonsense adjustments, but keep them within the basic framework of an age-appropriate schedule.

Position 1 Reminders

- Make sure your child gets good naps on the day of your first night of the Shuffle, according to the nap averages for your child's age in Chapter 2.

- Create your naptime, bedtime, and nighttime sleep plan on pages 80–83.

- Keep a sleep log.

- Plan an early enough bedtime. Watch her sleepy cues and the clock. Do the math backward. For example, a typical 1-year-old needs 11 to 11.5 hours of sleep at night. If her average wake-up time is 7 a.m., then she should be asleep by 7:30–8 p.m.

- Focus on what your plan is for the **first night**. Discuss it with her other parent to maintain a united front. Split the night up, take turns every other night, or decide who is going to get up for which awakenings.

- Drowsy but awake: That means more awake than drowsy. If you help your child get into a very drowsy state at bedtime, you'll make it harder for her to go back to sleep when she wakes during the night.

- Your child should be aware that she's being put down, which means she may cry, so be prepared.

- Your first chair position is **by the crib**.

- Be careful not to create a new sleep crutch. For example, don't substitute rocking your child to sleep with patting her back to sleep. Hint: You know you're patting too much if your child starts crying when you stop touching her.

- There is no limit to how long you sit by your child's bed. Stay as long as it takes, knowing that you don't want to train her to cry. You also don't want to sneak out too soon. When you do that your child (especially if she's over a year old) will become hypervigilant about your leaving, and will be up multiple times checking on you.

- Remember, you can pick your child up! You'll know within one to two nights whether it helps.

- Pick up to calm and *not to put to sleep*.

- Each time your child wakes up, go over to her crib: Figure out what she needs, encourage her to lie down, reassure her, and sit in your chair.

- Treat each night awakening the same (if you're not feeding during the night).

- Don't give up until after 6 a.m. Then do dramatic wake-up:

Leave the room, count to 10, and come back in as if nothing happened!

- Start nap coaching on day two.

- Remember, you can add additional nights if you need to. Try adding only one or two nights to each position and watch your child. Remember, the key is to keep moving incrementally, so that your child makes progress in learning the skill of putting herself to sleep. If you stay too long in one place, your child may simply have a new crutch.

POSITION 2

Move the chair about halfway to the door. (If the room is very small, or the crib is close to the door, you should skip to the next chair position and sit by the door in her room.) Continue the soothing sounds, but stay in the chair as much as you can. Get up to pat or stroke your child a little if necessary, or make the same soothing sounds as you have the past three nights. Try not to pick her up unless she's hysterical. Stay in the chair halfway to the door until she falls asleep.

When your child wakes up during the night, return to the chair position you were in at bedtime that night and soothe her. You can go over to her crib initially and quickly calm, caress, and encourage her to lie down (if she's standing or sitting) before you return to your chair by the door. Continue the soothing sounds but stay in the chair as much as you can. Get up to pat or stroke her a little if necessary. Try not to pick her up unless she's hysterical, and if you do pick her up, follow the technique described for the first three nights. Stay in your chair by the door until she's asleep again.

Position 2 Reminders

- There are still night awakenings, but you will have to move your **chair halfway to the door** on the fourth night.

- Keep a sleep log.

- Put your child into the crib drowsy but awake.

- You may get out of your chair and go to the crib to comfort your child if she becomes hysterical.

- Be careful about your child's efforts to get you to come to her— like throwing things out of her crib. Set a limit, such as "Lie down, sweetie, and Mommy will get you your binky. But you must lie down." You also may have to limit how many times you will return it. Follow through on whatever you say.

- It's common to see a regression the first night you move your chair farther away.

- Children get ritualized easily. Make changes every three to five days, if at all possible. Look back at "When—and How—to Slow Things Down" in Chapter 3 if you need help with the schedule.

- The first night in a new position may be the hardest. Stay the course!

POSITION 3

Move the **chair to the doorway or the doorjamb inside her room**. You should be in dim light but still visible. Continue the same soothing techniques from your chair, remembering to intervene as little as possible. Don't worry if she cries a bit; keep quietly reassuring her. She'll know you're there, and she'll fall asleep.

When your child wakes up during the night, return to the chair position you were in at bedtime that night and soothe her. You can go over to the crib initially and quickly calm and caress her, and then encourage her to lie down (if she's standing or sitting) before you return to your chair by the door. Continue the soothing sounds, but stay in the chair as much as you can. Get up to pat or stroke her a little, if necessary. Try not to pick her up unless she's hysterical, and if you do pick her up, follow the technique described for the first three nights. Stay in your chair by the door until she falls back to sleep.

Position 3 Reminders

- On night seven you will move your **chair to the door inside the room**.

- Use your voice to reassure her.

- Keep a sleep log.

- You may get out of your chair and go to the crib to comfort your child if she becomes hysterical.

- For all nighttime awakenings, you can go to the crib initially, see what your child needs, encourage her to lie down, reassure her, and then go back to your chair by the door.

- If you are adding one or two nights on to each position, continue with the plan. Do not add additional nights at this time; continue with the number of nights you set as your goal.

POSITION 4

Move the **chair to the hallway, with the door open enough so your child can still see you from the crib**. The hall should be dimly lit. Stay until she falls asleep.

When your child wakes up during the night, return to the chair position you were in at bedtime that night and soothe her. You can go over to the crib initially and quickly calm and caress her, and encourage her to lie down (if she's standing or sitting) before you return to your chair by the door. Continue the soothing sounds, but stay in the chair as much as you can. Get up to pat or stroke her a little if necessary. Try not to pick her up unless she's hysterical, and if you do pick her up, follow the technique described for the first three nights. Stay in your chair in the hallway in view until she's asleep.

Position 4 Reminders

- Your new chair position on night 10 is the **hallway in view**.

- Your child's bedroom door should be open enough for her to see you from her crib.

- Keep a sleep log.

- This next move on the first night can be difficult because you're not in the room and your child may try every trick she can think of to get you back there. She may throw things or cry until you come; if she's verbal, she might even kick off her blanket and then call you to tuck her back in. Set a limit such as "Mommy will only tuck you in one more time and then you will have to do it yourself." Follow through on whatever you say.

- If you've been consistent until now you will probably begin to see some improvement—such as fewer, shorter night awakenings. Congratulations!

- With consistency on your part, night sleep can fall into place as soon as 7 to 10 nights for children up to age 18 months, and in 2 to 3 weeks in children over 18 months. Naps for children with special needs often become much more organized and stable within 2 to 3 weeks. Afternoon naps and early rising can take as long as 3 to 4 weeks to improve.

POSITION 5

By now your child is probably falling asleep and staying asleep on her own. Your last step is to give her a chance to do this without you there at all. It may seem like a huge leap, but it's not so big for her. After all, she's had nearly two weeks of preparation! Move farther down the hall, so that you're **out of view but your child can hear you**. You can keep making "sh-sh" sounds—not constantly, but often enough to let her know that you're close by and responsive. If she cries,

check on her from the door—don't go to her crib. Be calm and reassuring. Make some comforting, encouraging sounds to convey that
you're not far away and that you know she can put herself to sleep.
Your child really can soothe herself to sleep—if you give her the opportunity.

Position 5 Reminders

- It's okay to break up this step if it's very upsetting to your child.
  For instance, you could sit halfway out of view the first night
  and then move to totally out of view a night or two later.

- Night awakenings have greatly diminished by now and you may
  only be struggling with early rising. This is especially true if your
  child had a previous history of early rising. Stay consistent and
  work on those naps. Early rising can take three to four weeks
  to improve!

- Remember that early rising is caused by one or more of the following:

  - a too-late bedtime;

  - nap deprivation in general;

  - a too-large wake-up window between afternoon nap and
    bedtime. This window should not exceed four hours for a
    child who is not sleeping through the night yet.

  - putting your child to bed too drowsy at bedtime.

The two hardest parts of sleep coaching are early rising and the
stubborn afternoon naps. Stay consistent and these will improve!

CHAPTER TWELVE

Implementing Your Plan for a Child in a Bed

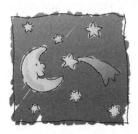 A child who's old enough to sleep in a big-kid bed is old enough to become invested in improving his own sleep and can feel proud when he does. Positive reinforcement goes a long way for this age group.

Children who move from the crib too early don't necessarily have the verbal skills to understand big-boy or big-girl bedtime rules. These skills develop around 2½ years old for neurotypical children, so it is best to have your child with special needs sleep in a crib as long as possible. If your child is already in a bed, but moved too early, this process may take longer and you may very well have to install a gate. Be patient and consistent. If your toddler is on a mattress on the floor or in a low toddler bed, sit nearby on the floor, not on a chair.

THE FAMILY MEETING

If you've found your child responds well to having a short discussion and a chance to ask questions about changes to his routine or usual schedule, hold a short family meeting before beginning sleep coaching. Choose a time when your child is happy and receptive. Sunday morning after pancakes is a lot better than 5 p.m. on a weekday on which he skipped his nap and is starving for dinner. Tell him that you read a book by The Sleep Lady and learned about how children can sleep better. That way you can blame me for any changes or rules

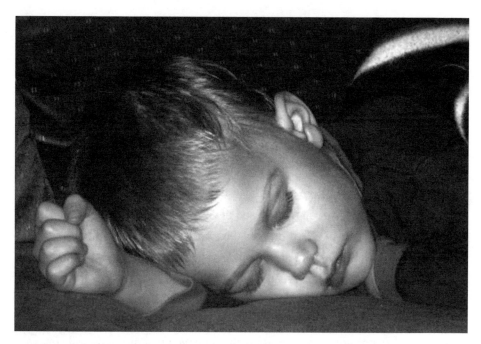

Kaden, age 3½

he doesn't like. For instance, if your child begs you to lie down with him you can tell him The Sleep Lady said we can't do that but we can stay with you in your room. Some children get furious. "The Sleep Lady can't come over to play with me!" "I don't like The Sleep Lady." But when they succeed, when they start feeling good about their new sleep skills, they often want to call me on the phone and tell me how proud they are of themselves! In the back of this workbook is a certificate you can tear out, fill in, and give to your child!

Keep the discussion upbeat and positive. You don't want your child to feel he has a problem or that he's doing something wrong. Portray it as your problem, your responsibility. "Mommy and Daddy should have helped you learn to put yourself to sleep sooner and we are sorry we didn't. But The Sleep Lady helped us understand that and now we are going to help you learn." Explain that children who go to bed without fussing, and who sleep all night, feel better in the morning and have more fun during the day. Encourage your child to brainstorm about how he can participate, maybe by deciding what he can take into his bed to touch or hug, what pictures should be taken for his Sleep Story, or what extra game he will get to play in the morning if he uses good sleep manners at night. You want him to have a stake in success. You may be surprised at how sensitive children already are to sleep issues and how quickly they pick up the lingo. Many kids are relieved when parents bring this up. They know that something is wrong, that Mom and Dad are frustrated and want them to sleep differently. They're happy to know you are going to help them.

If you think it will be useful, you can give your child examples, preferably of an older friend or cousin he looks up to. Say something like, "We're going to teach you how to put yourself to sleep and to sleep all night long in your own bed, just like cousin Johnny and cousin Jenny and Gramma and Aunt Rachel." Be sure to frame this in a positive way, not one to make your child feel ashamed.

Explain clearly and specifically what changes are coming: "Daddy is not going to lie down with you anymore, but Daddy will stay with you until you fall asleep." Or, "If you come to our bed at night, we're going to tell you we love you and take you back into your bed where you can snuggle with your teddy bear." Adapt the script to the appropriate sleep challenge but don't give too much detail. You can introduce the idea of a sticker chart so your child will know exactly what behavior you'll expect.

THE SLEEP LADY SHUFFLE FOR CHILDREN IN A BED

It's not as easy to do the Shuffle with a child in a bed as it is with an infant in a crib. Even though the Shuffle is gentle and gradual, older children still get upset and fight the change. If you've got a little resister on your hands don't get angry, but don't give up either. Keep reminding him that he can learn to put himself to sleep in his "big boy" bed without Mommy lying down with him.

Throughout the Shuffle we try to minimize tears, but we can't promise to eliminate them completely. To keep the tears in check, give lots of reassurance, lots of love, and lots of praise. In addition to reviewing rules and expectations every night at bedtime, you should also pay your child sleep compliments during the day.

POSITION 1

Once bath, stories, songs, and review of his sleep manners are over, **sit in a chair or on the floor next to your child's bed**. Stroke or pat him intermittently if he fusses or cries, but don't do it constantly or he'll form a new negative association and will need you to pat him constantly in order to fall asleep. Likewise, don't let him hold your hand: You should control all physical contact. You can be a little more generous with touch the first night, when the whole system is new to him, but be careful about creating difficult new patterns, starting on the second night.

Your child will almost certainly try to engage you. **Try closing your eyes**, which not only conveys an unambiguous message that it's time to sleep, but also makes it easier for you to resist getting drawn into a conversation or philosophical discussion about the nature of the universe. **Stay there until he falls asleep**.

Some children get quite upset if you won't lie down with them. In desperation their parents might put their head down on the pillow next to their child. Try not to do it, but if you do, please limit it to the first night or you aren't going to make much progress. You won't be teaching him new skills if you're sharing a pillow!

Close your eyes and "sh-sh" him. If he continues to reach for you, then you may have to scoot your chair away from the bed a bit so you have to lean in to touch him.

Remember, in three more nights you won't be sitting next to him and won't be able to touch him constantly. You want to be able to fade out of his sleep picture, not add to his fury with every change.

Each time your child wakes during the night respond to him the same way. If he calls for you from his bed or gets out of bed and comes to your room, take his hand and walk him back to his bed. If using one, remind him that his clock has not turned colors yet and that he needs to lie quietly in his bed and go back to sleep. Sit quietly in your chair by his bed until he does.

Position 1 Reminders

- Wake your child if he's not awake by 7:30 a.m. the morning of the day you'll begin sleep coaching.

- Make sure your child gets a good nap on the day of the first night of the Shuffle.

- Create your nap, bedtime, and nighttime sleep plans on pages 80–83.

- Create your sleep manners chart.

- Create a routine checklist.

- Create your Sleep Story.

- Purchase and set up your wake-up clock, if using (see page 132 for suggestions).

- Keep a sleep log.

- Have your family meeting before bedtime.

- Plan an early enough bedtime.

- Your first chair position is by the bed.

- There is no time limit on how long you sit by your child at bed-time while he goes to sleep. Minimize your interactions.

- Remember, you can hug your child if he gets really worked up! Just don't lie down with him or cuddle him until he goes to sleep.

- Encourage him to pull up his blankets, find his lovey or pacifier, or have a sip of his water by himself.

- Treat each night awakening the same. If your child calls for you from his bed or gets out of bed and comes to your room, take his hand and walk him back to his bed. Remind him that his clock has not turned colors yet and that he needs to lie quietly in his bed and go back to sleep. Sit quietly in your chair until he does.

- Don't give up until after 6 a.m.! Wait until your child's wake-up music or light comes on and then do a dramatic wake-up: leave the room, count to 10, and then come back in as if nothing happened. And remember, if you allow your child to get out of bed and start his day before the wake-up music comes on, then he won't take it seriously. After all, you're not, so why should he?

- Each morning, go over your child's sleep manners chart before or during breakfast. Make sure you have his attention (the TV should be off) and give him stickers or stars to reward him for when he did a good job. Talk to him about the behaviors you want to see more of.

- Start nap coaching on day two if you are going to start both elements of coaching at the same time.

- Remember, you can extend this one to two extra nights. You want to find a balance between moving regularly to teach your child the skill of falling asleep independently, while making sure that he feels supported along the way. More important, you want to strike this balance without creating another sleep crutch (i.e., he now needs you to be sitting in a chair next to his bed every time he goes to sleep and multiple times throughout the night).

POSITION 2

Children with special needs often do better when they know what to expect. They also respond well to positive reinforcement. Tell your child what a good job he's been doing and that you're going to move your chair. Remind him that you'll still stay in the room until he falls asleep. **Move the chair to the door.**

You may occasionally "sh-sh" if needed, but stay as quiet as you can. Explain to your child that once the lights are out, there's no more talking.

If he gets really upset and you feel he needs help calming down, then go to his bedside, reassure him, and give him a hug. Remind him that you aren't going to leave him and that you'll stay until he falls asleep. Don't let him fall asleep in your arms or on your lap and don't lie down with him. Keep telling him what a good job he's doing, and how proud you are of him.

Your child may get out of bed and come to your chair. He may try to bring you back to his bed or crawl into your lap. Give him a big hug and tell him that if he'll get back into his bed by himself, you'll come over and tuck him in. If he does it a second or third time, tell him this will be the last time you'll tuck him in.

By this point, most kids get tired and stay in bed, especially if they're getting the message that Mom or Dad is going to stick around until they fall asleep. But if your child doesn't stop getting out of bed, stand up and explain clearly that if he keeps it up, you will have to leave. Say something like, "If you don't follow your sleep manners and lie quietly in your bed, then I'm going to have to leave your room." If that doesn't work, there are a couple of things you can try:

- Put a gate in the doorway and sit on the other side of it. Let your child know that if he gets into bed and stays there, you'll come in and tuck him in. If he nods off on the floor near the gate, move him when he's in a sound sleep.

- Stand up and tell your child that if he doesn't get into bed and lie quietly you will leave and close the door. Count to three and give him one more chance to get back in bed. If he doesn't, leave the room, close the door, and stand on the other side of the door and count to three again. Open the door and say calmly, "Get back into your bed and I will come sit in your room." Chances are he'll hop right into bed because he wants you in the room. Some children will test a parent to see if they'll follow through on the threat, though; if that happens, count to three again, leave the room, close the door, and so on. Some parents have to do this a few times before their child takes them seriously and stays in bed.

Each time your child wakes during the night, respond to him the same way. If he calls for you from his bed or gets out of bed and comes to your room, take his hand and walk him back to bed. If he calls from the gate, tell him you will come tuck him in if he gets back into bed on his own. Remind him that his wake-up music or light is not on yet and that he needs to lie quietly in his bed and go back to sleep. Sit quietly in your chair by the door until he does. Take a look back at the visual supports in Chapter 6 if you need help with this.

Position 2 Reminders

- Your chair position is **in the room by the door**.

- Review your child's sleep manners chart and read his Sleep Story at bedtime.

- Use the routine checklist for the bedtime routine.

- Keep a sleep log.

- It is common to see a regression the first night you move your chair farther away.

- There are still night awakenings, but do not wait too many more nights; try to move within three to five days.

- You may get out of your chair and go to your child's bedside to comfort him if he becomes hysterical. Don't stay too long and create a new crutch, such as patting him back to sleep. It happens easily!

- Be careful about how you respond to your child's efforts to get you to come to his bedside—such as kicking off his blankets and asking you to cover him back up. Put a limit on the number of times you'll comply: "Only two cover ups, honey." Encourage your child to pull up his own blankets, find his lovey or pacifier, or have a sip of his water (put it in a cup where he can reach it) by himself.

• Treat each night awakening the same. If your child calls for you from his bed or gets out of bed and comes to your room, take his hand and walk him back to his room. Remind him that his wake-up music or light is not on yet and that he needs to lie quietly in bed and go back to sleep. Sit in your chair by the door until he's back asleep.

• Don't give up until after 6 a.m.! Wait until the wake-up music comes on and then do a dramatic wake-up: Leave the room, count to 10, and come back in as if nothing happened.

• Each morning, review your child's sleep manners chart before or during breakfast. Make sure you have his attention (no TV), and give him stickers or stars for when he did a good job. Focus on the behavior you want to see more of and let your child know he can do it. If helpful, call a loved one who lives far away, or tell his teachers about his progress to encourage and motivate your child.

POSITION 3

Tell your child that he's doing a great job and explain that you're going to move the chair again. Show him where it will be—**in the hallway where he can see you from his bed**. Continue the same soothing techniques, intervening as little as possible. He may cry a bit but gently reassure him and he will fall asleep. If he keeps getting out of bed and coming to you, tell him you will come tuck him in, but he must first get back in bed by himself. If he lies down on the floor, ignore it. Move him to his bed if he falls asleep.

If he continues to get out of bed and come to you in the hallway, consider installing a gate (if you haven't already). Explain to your child that the gate is there to help him remember his sleep manners and to stay quietly in his bed. Add that once he remembers all his sleep manners for a whole week (at least), you will take the gate down. Make sure you also explain to him that he may not climb the gate since that is very dangerous. (You'll be sitting right by the gate so you'll also be able to catch any climbing attempts.)

If you do put up a gate, sit on the other side of it at bedtime and for all night awakenings. Don't climb over the gate to hug or reassure your child until he gets back in bed himself. If you haven't gated your child's door and he comes into your room, take his hand and walk him back to his own room. Remind him that his wake-up music or light is not on yet and he needs to lie quietly in bed and go back to sleep. Tuck him in and sit in your chair in the hall until he's asleep.

Position 3 Reminders

- Move your chair to the **hallway where your child can see you from his bed**.

- Use your voice to reassure him.

- Review your child's sleep manners chart and read his Sleep Story at bedtime.

- Use the routine checklist for the bedtime routine.

- Keep a sleep log.

- The move to the hallway can be difficult because you're no longer in the room. Your child may try every trick he can think of to get you back in, including crying, throwing things, or kicking off the blankets and begging to be tucked back in. Set a limit such as "Mommy will only tuck you in one more time and then you will have to do it yourself." Follow through on whatever you say.

If your child starts to display unsafe behavior (hitting his head or body or other self-injurious behavior), set up the bed and bedroom with as many soft surfaces as possible. Line the edges of the bed with blankets or pads. If your child is still unsafe or hurting himself, silently walk into the room, go to his bed, and say "It's night time" or any other phrase you have been using during sleep coaching. Encourage your child to lie down by patting the mattress. Once he has calmed a bit, you can give him a quick hug or kiss, reiterate that it is bedtime, and return to your place. You may have to do this a few times. Remain calm (it can be difficult) and neutral so that your child sees that you are not going to stop everything; you are going to encourage him to be safe, and try again.

- Treat each night awakening the same. If you haven't gated your child's door and he calls for you from his bed or comes into your room, take his hand and walk him back to his own room. Remind him that his wake-up music is not on yet and he needs to lie quietly in bed and go back to sleep. Tuck him in and sit in your chair in the hall until he's asleep.

- If he calls out during the night and there's a gate in his doorway, go to the gate, point out that his wake-up music or light isn't on, and tell him that you'll come into his room and tuck him in if he gets into bed by himself and stays there. If he conks out on the floor near the gate, move him later, when he's sound asleep.

- Don't give up until after 6 a.m. Wait until the wake-up music comes on and then do a dramatic wake-up. If you're already sitting in the hall from an early rising, acknowledge that the wake-up music has now come on and it's time to get up. Remember, if you allow your child to get out of bed before his music comes on, he won't take the music seriously.

- Each morning, review your child's sleep manners chart with him before or during breakfast. Make sure you have his attention (no TV), and give him stickers or stars for doing a good job. Focus on the behavior you want to see more of.

POSITION 4

Move a few feet farther down the hallway, so that you're **out of sight but within hearing distance**. Make "sh-sh" sounds from the hallway, just frequently enough that your child knows you're near. If he gets up to look for you, take him back to bed. If you haven't already, put a gate in his doorway if he gets up excessively.

Take this step slowly if it really upsets your child. For instance, you can sit halfway out of view and then move completely out of view one or two nights later.

If your child calls for you from his bed or gets out of bed during the night (if you haven't gated his door) and comes to your room, take his hand and walk him back to his room. Point out that his wake-up music or light isn't on yet and tell him he needs to go back to sleep. Tuck him in and sit quietly in your chair in the hall until he's back asleep. If your child's sleep has improved sufficiently by now (he's waking up less often and for shorter periods) and his room is close enough to yours, you can also try going back to your bed right away and reassuring him from there. If he calls out during the night and you have installed a gate, go to the gate, remind him that his wake-up music or light is not on yet, and tell him you'll come and tuck him in if he gets back in bed and stays there. If he falls asleep on the floor near the gate, move him later when he's sound asleep.

Position 4 Reminders

- Your chair position is in the **hallway out of view**.

- Use your voice to reassure your child if needed. Do not shush, talk, or sing constantly up until the time your child is asleep.

- Review your child's sleep manners chart at bedtime, and read his Sleep Story.

- Use the bedtime checklist during the bedtime routine.

- Keep a sleep log.

- If your child comes to his doorway to check that you're in the hall as promised, but then gets right back into bed by himself, ignore it.

- Treat each night awakening the same. If your child calls from his bed during the night or gets out of bed and comes to your room, take his hand and walk him back to his room. Point out that his wake-up music isn't on yet and tell him to go back to sleep. Tuck him in and sit quietly in your chair in the hall (or go back to your own bed if your room is close enough, and reassure him from there).

- If he calls out during the night and you have installed a gate, go to the gate, remind him that his wake-up music or light is not on yet, and tell him you'll come tuck him in if he gets back into bed and stays there. If he falls asleep on the floor near the gate, move him after he's sound asleep.

- Don't give up until after 6 a.m. Then, when the wake-up music comes on, do dramatic wake-up: If you're already in the hall from an earlier rising, acknowledge that the wake-up music has now come on and that it's time to start the day. Remember, if you allow your child to get out of bed before the music comes on, he won't take it seriously.

- Each morning, review your child's sleep manners chart before or during breakfast. Make sure you have his attention (no TV), give him stickers or stars for his chart, and focus on the behaviors you want to see more of.

- If you've been consistent, by now the night awakenings should be greatly diminished and you may only be struggling with early rising. This is especially true if your child has a previous history of early rising. Early rising can take three to four weeks to improve!

Remember that early rising is caused by one or more of the following:

- a too-late bedtime;

- nap deprivation in general;

- too much time between the end of the afternoon nap and bedtime (average window is four to five hours for a well-rested child);

- putting your child to bed too drowsy at bedtime.

POSITION 5

A fair number of children start falling asleep and staying asleep between nights 10 and 14—occasionally even sooner. But most parents have to take one more step: Put away the chair and leave their child alone for five-minute intervals, or what we call "job checks." To do this, tell your child that you will keep checking on him from his doorway until he's asleep.

Most likely your child won't have a realistic concept of how long five minutes is. It may sound like a very long time, so explain exactly what you'll be doing and where you'll be during that time (brushing your teeth in the bathroom, changing clothes in your bedroom, folding laundry in the living room). Always return as promised and check on him from his doorway.

By now your child has had weeks of preparation. He has given up some of his negative associations and gained quite a bit of sleep independence. Don't go too far away—stay on the same floor, in a nearby room, and read a magazine or a book for the first few nights. Gradually, you can move a little farther away. If he cries, you'll be back every five minutes to reassure him. Try not to go to the door more than that; he'll get more stimulated and more upset if he has to say goodbye to you every two minutes.

Unlike the crying-it-out approach to sleep coaching, you don't need to keep stretching out the intervals for longer than five minutes. The only exception is if you sense that five minutes is too brief for your child, and that having to see you but separate again every five minutes is making him more agitated. Then experiment and see if he finds it less disturbing if you check on him every 10 or 15 minutes.

CHAPTER THIRTEEN

Troubleshooting

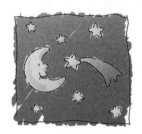

1. **My daughter likes to play with my hair during the entire bedtime routine until she falls asleep. How can I break this habit?**

Many children, whether or not they have a specific diagnosis, engage in stereotypical and/or ritualization behaviors. In this workbook, we're talking about behaviors that are usually repetitive, such as (but not limited to) lining up toys or items in bed, making noises over and over again, twirling someone else's hair, and so forth.

It's important to put limits on these behaviors and to then reward a child who stays within those limits. For instance, if her sleep crutch is twirling a parent's hair, first make clear when and for how long she's allowed to do it: "You can twirl my hair gently during story time, but when the story is finished, it will be time to stop twirling my hair." Make this an item on her sleep manners chart, as well as a "no more twirling" on her visual schedule for the bedtime routine. Follow through with praise and appropriate rewards (a sticker on her manners chart, for example).

For a kid who lines toys up on her bed and can't relax or focus on anything else, it may be helpful to simply remove the items. Offer lots of support, though: Talk to her about it if she is developmentally able to understand and link the limits you're making on lining up the items to her sleep manners chart. You might also find something else for her to focus on that's more appropriate for bedtime, such as a lovey. The only danger here is the lovey could become another crutch; if that happens you'll have to take it away too, until you've established healthy sleep habits without it. Then you may be able to re-introduce a lovey or even the items she likes to line up.

Another way to set limits on a ritualized behavior is by setting a timer. Explain in clear language what will happen when it goes off: "Now it's time to line up your toys. When the timer goes off, we'll turn the lights off." Be consistent about setting the timer, not negotiating for extra time, or allowing your child to engage you in arguments or conversation. This way she doesn't have to give up the activity, but there also are reasonable boundaries around it that she can understand. Again, this can be a sleep manners item on her chart.

2. My toddler has started banging his head against the crib rails at bedtime.

If your child expresses frustration, anxiety, or anger by banging his head or otherwise causing pain, he may resort to such behavior during the Shuffle.

Try not to be alarmed and certainly don't give up sleep coaching. Instead, take time to figure out why your child is engaging in the behavior so you can come up with a way to stop him from hurting himself. Remember, behavior is a form of communication. Your child is trying to tell you something. He may be banging his head for sensory reasons: It actually feels good.

On the other hand, he may be feeling confused or frustrated with the process of sleep coaching and finds it easier or more effective to use this behavior to convey that message. He knows that if he engages in an alarming behavior, his parent is likely to rush to his rescue and even toss the entire sleep-coaching process out the window in order to make him stop.

How can you sleep coach your child and keep him safe at the same time? Whether he's hurting himself because it feels good or he's trying to distract from the coaching process (and get your attention), your first step is to set up his sleeping space so that it's soft and there are no exposed corners or rails. You can purchase vertical crib liners (see page 133) or, if your child is in a bed, wrap all sharp edges and corners with blankets or towels. If there are objects in your child's bed that he's using for self-injurious behavior, remove them before bedtime.

If the behavior seems sensory in nature, ask your child's team to suggest sensory-based strategies to add to the bedtime routine that might safely meet his sensory needs. His occupational therapist, if he has one, may be particularly helpful in this area.

But if you suspect your child is causing himself pain because he's frustrated, tell him "no" as calmly but firmly as you can when he starts the behavior. Tell him to lie down or pat the mattress to encourage him to lie down. Once he does, pat or stroke him, tell him you love him, and then go back to your coaching position. You may have to do this many times in the beginning. Try not to give him extra attention, physical contact, or time sitting next to him. Be consistent. Once your child learns that his behavior ultimately won't stop the coaching, he's likely to stop doing it. Remember, with any change in behavior things often get worse before they get better. Stay the course.

3. My child has been throwing a fit at bedtime ever since we started the Shuffle.

It's not unusual for kids to have tantrums at bedtime. First, make sure your child isn't over-tired. When you ask an exhausted kid to do anything—from brushing her teeth to getting into bed—she may have a tantrum. Time your evenings well to support your child's needs, especially in those first days of the Shuffle.

Even if you time it perfectly, your child may resist every step of the bedtime routine or maybe one part in particular. Either way, continue as calmly and neutrally as you can. Make it clear that the process will continue no matter how much she acts up. You can empathize by saying "I know it's hard," or using other simple language, but don't get caught up in a full-blown lecture or conversation. And don't feel guilty: You have set up a supportive and reasonable routine for your child and you aren't asking her to do something she can't do. You're also making it clear that you're there to help her with the challenging parts.

Refer to the strategies in Chapter 5 and the visuals in Chapter 6 to try to nip tantrums in the bud before they even start. Offer your child reasonable choices along the way: For example, let her decide if she wants to brush her teeth before she puts on her pajamas or after. (But of course, don't make either of those steps optional!) Having some degree of control over the routine will make it more acceptable to your child.

Note, too, that tantrums often are a response to change, so once your child gets used to the new approach to bedtime, she'll be less likely to resist. Your job is to be consistent. Stick with it.

4. I need to coach a baby and a toddler who sleep in separate bedrooms. Is that even possible?

Absolutely—especially if there are two parents or caregivers on hand at bedtime. Before you start, wait for an evening (or ideally a few evenings in a row) when you and your spouse or partner will both be home at bedtime or recruit a friend or family member. One adult puts the baby to sleep and the other puts the toddler to sleep using the Shuffle techniques. If you have to go it alone, start with the baby. Set up the older child with a quiet activity while you do the Shuffle with the little one, and then move on to sleep coaching the toddler.

5. I'm worried that the child I'm sleep coaching will wake my other kid. What then?

This is a common concern. Many parents will rush in to soothe one child to avoid disturbing the other. Try not to fall into this trap: It will only perpetuate one child's night awakenings by reinforcing one or both children's sleep crutches. If one child wakes the other, then start with the older child. For instance, if you're working with a 6-month-old and she wakes up a 2-year-old in the process, go to the toddler, reassure him that the baby is okay, and tell him he can go back to sleep—then tend to the baby. If there are two adults in the house, then divide and conquer, one of you with each child. Try not to panic and start any negative habits with your toddler that you'll have to change, such as lying down with him to get him back to sleep quickly and quietly. We also recommend putting a white noise machine in an older child's room to mask the sound of other things going on the house (some favorites are listed in Chapter 15), or you could use a fan.

6. My children share a room. How do I sleep coach them?

There are several possible scenarios here:

- If your children already share a room, move one of them out temporarily—to a makeshift bed in your room, for example, or a spare bedroom if you have one—until the other is consistently sleeping through the night. This option can work very well if the child who moves already has good sleep habits. Explain to her that this arrangement is temporary— just until her little brother or sister learns how to sleep well. When it's time for her to move back into the shared room, make clear that she mustn't talk to or play with her sibling—that everyone needs to be sleeping. Explain that sharing a room is special and it's important to have good "sleep manners."
- If you're sleep coaching two children with special needs at once who share a room (whether they're in beds or cribs), you can work with both at the same time. Sit between the beds or cribs and alternately comfort each child according to the Shuffle technique. If two adults are available, each can "take a child" for the crib-side/bedside position. Only one parent is necessary for the subsequent chair positions.

7. Should I tell my older child that I will be sleep coaching her sibling?

Certainly. Explain what's going on and help her feel like she's a part of it. Depending on her age and sleep skills, you may even help her think of herself as a sleep role model for the sibling. Tell her that her brother needs to know how to get himself to sleep, just like she does. Explain that when he learns, he won't cry as much, but in the meantime, you have to be with him or check on him frequently. The older child will let you go more easily if you make her an ally.

8. What if my child gets sick in the middle of sleep training?

Don't abandon the program completely: If you can, maintain your Shuffle position until he's better. If you feel he absolutely needs you closer, go back to sitting near his crib or bed as you did on the first three nights of the Shuffle, and then move to the door when he is feeling better. Don't draw this out or you will just make it harder for him. If he gets sick shortly after you complete his coaching, he'll probably backslide a bit and you may have to do an abbreviated version of the Shuffle to get him sleeping all night again.

When your child is sick, respond immediately to his cries at night and do whatever you need to do—give him medicine, aspirate his nose, clean him up after a tummy attack. Hold and comfort him as much as you think he needs, even if it sets back sleep training a few days. Soothe and take care of your child, but try not to totally regress.

9. My child consistently wakes up before 6 a.m. What's going on?

It's likely your child is getting to bed too late, getting too little sleep during the day, is awake for too long between her afternoon nap and bedtime, or is being put down already asleep at bedtime. Check with your pediatrician to rule out any underlying medical causes that could be contributing to the early rising, such as obstructive sleep apnea. Check your sleep log to make sure she's getting enough daytime sleep and going to bed early enough and awake enough to really master the skill of putting herself to sleep. Children 5 years and under should generally be going to bed between 7 p.m. and 8 p.m.

If your child has been getting up and staying up earlier than 6 a.m. for several months, you have an established pattern that will probably take three to four weeks to change.

You will have to work on naps and bedtime at the same time as the early-morning awakenings.

- Put up room-darkening shades. This alone can make a big difference.

- When your child wakes up, go in initially at, say, 5 a.m. and tell her, "It's not time to get up." Point out that the wake-up music or light isn't on (if you're using either of them). Depending on your child's age, you might say, "Mommy and Daddy are sleeping."

- If you're in the process of the Shuffle, then after your brief initial check resume your chair position until the wake-up music or light comes on.

- If you believe that staying in your child's room during these early risings is keeping her up, consider leaving. In that case, when she wakes up, go into her room, remind her about the wake-up music, offer her lovey and verbal and physical reassurance, and then leave the room. Make your visit brief so as not to further awaken her. Go in for brief checks every 15 to 20 minutes until 6 a.m., when you make it your final visit. At that point go into the room and say, "Good morning! Your wake-up music is on." Perform a "dramatic wake-up": Excitedly open the shades and get your child up to start the day. Don't talk about or refer to your earlier visits. With this routine, you're conveying the following message to your child: "Getting you out of bed has nothing to do with how long you have been crying—it's because it is *time* to get up."

A toddler clock often is easy enough for a child to understand. Remind her that she must stay in bed until the music or light comes on.

10. Couldn't I fix the early-rising problem by simply putting my child to bed later?

Unfortunately, no! The only time that might work is if the following apply:

- Your child is taking "good naps" (based on his age).

- Your child appears rested and happy during the day with less than the average night's sleep for the child's age group.

- Your child consistently sleeps through the night and is not off the sleep average by more than one hour.

- You child seems rested and ready to start his day at 6 a.m. and can make it to naptime without getting too sleepy.

11. My child soaks through her diapers at night. What should I do?

Try using extra-absorbent overnight diapers or a larger-size diaper with an insert, or "doubler"—a pad that you can stick in the diaper. They can be handy on long car or plane trips as well. If you have to change your child's diaper and you're fast at it, you might be able to remove a soaked diaper quickly without taking her out of her crib or bed. If your child is 3 or older, talk to your pediatrician to rule out sleep apnea, which can increase bedwetting.

12. My child poops every time I put him in his crib. What should I do?

Some children dirty their diaper just as you put them to bed at night or naptime—and some parents become convinced it's intentional, that the child knows you will pick him up and get him out of the crib. Obviously, you need to change the diaper, but do it as quietly as you can, in light as dim as possible. If you can manage it, change him in the bed or crib and then hand him his lovey and return to your Shuffle position. If this happens at naptime, change him, but approach it as a too-short nap and follow the nap-training advice in Chapter 7. If it happens at 5 a.m., change him and follow the advice for early risers. Children often have a hard time going back to sleep after a 30-minute nap and then a diaper change, or after a 5 a.m. diaper change. You may see some crying, but be consistent and reassuring. If you have completed the Shuffle and you feel your child needs a little more reassurance than normal to go back to sleep after his diaper change, then it's okay to sit closer that night if you feel it will help. On the following night, return to your usual routine.

13. My child vomits when I put her into her crib. What should I do?

A lot of parents worry that if they let their babies cry too long, the child will vomit, particularly if she has or had reflux. This may be the case if you leave a child to cry on her own, but it seldom happens when the parent remains in the room and practices my gentler, more gradual method. To alleviate this problem, don't feed your child right before sleep.

Some children vomit on purpose because they know the parent will take them out of their crib and fuss over them. If you see your child trying to make herself gag (some kids can do this without using fingers!), firmly say, "No!" but immediately follow up with soothing reassurance. If she does throw up, clean up quickly and engage with her as little as possible. Use wipes or a washcloth, if you can, rather than getting her completely up for a bath. Don't turn the lights on. Some parents leave an extra sheet on the floor for children who tend to vomit over the crib railing. This makes cleanup easier since they can just roll it up and toss it in the hamper. Then reassure your child back to sleep. Remember, you don't want to give the message that if she throws up she will get out of the crib and not have to go to sleep.

Obviously, this doesn't apply to a child who is sick. In that case, you need to comfort her and follow your doctor's timetable for giving her fluids.

14. My child can't seem to settle down at all when I sit by his crib. What do I do?

If you're absolutely convinced after at least four days of sitting in your child's room that your presence is overstimulating to him or you find it so hard to do it yourself that you can't be consistent, then we suggest you either have the other parent try or you leave the room and do timed checks. There is no magic rule about how often you check or how many times you check, and you may have to experiment a bit. If you check on him too soon, he may treat it like a game and get even more stimulated. If you are away too long, he may get himself worked up and upset. We suggest starting with every seven minutes and gradually increasing it, but trust your own instincts and make necessary adjustments; this isn't a one-size-fits-all approach. When you check on him, go right into the room to his crib. Give him a quick reassuring pat, but don't linger. You will defeat the whole purpose if you stand there for a half hour patting him to sleep.

Here's another variant: Sometimes the Shuffle works at night but not for naps when the child is more awake and more likely to keep trying to engage you. So feel free to stick to the Shuffle at night and use the timed checks described for the naps, if that's what feels right to you.

If your child is in a bed and continuously engaging with you sitting by the bed, move your chair and sit by the door before moving to timed checks. Timed checks with children in beds tends to lead to the child leaving the room several times, and multiple returns to bed can often lead to a full meltdown.

15. We live in a one-bedroom apartment and our toddler, who is in a crib, sleeps in the same room as we do. Can we do this while sleep training?

You can! Your chair positions at bedtime can be the same as those outlined in this workbook except for the middle of the night after night four. When your child wakes up during the night after your first three nights by the crib, go to the crib side to do an initial reassuring check and then return to your bed and use your voice to soothe your child. You could sit up in your bed so she can easily see you.

Some other tricks:

- Put the crib right next to your bed and then move it away at the beginning of the Shuffle.

- Use a screen or create a makeshift wall from a curtain tacked to the ceiling.

CHAPTER FOURTEEN

Sleep Log,
Sleep Manners Chart,
Sleep Story,
Bedtime Checklist and Pass,
and Award of Achievement

You can use the templates included in the following pages, or you can also go to www.sleeplady.com to download electronic templates that you can customize and use in your home.

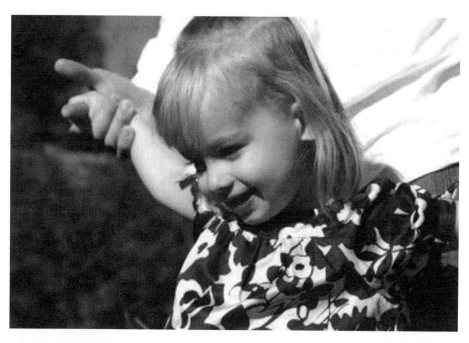

Emmalee, age 3½

Sleep Log

ACTIVITY (meal, nap, bed)	WHAT HAPPENED	AWAKE/ START	ASLEEP TIME	TOTAL TIME
Bedtime	Nursed well; cried on and off; picked up once	7:00 p.m.	7:30 p.m.	
Woke	Nursed well; cried on and off; picked up once	3:00 a.m.	3:40 a.m.	
Woke	Whimpered	5:40 a.m.	Dramatic wake-up at 6:00 a.m.	

Sleep Log

ACTIVITY (meal, nap, bed)	WHAT HAPPENED	AWAKE/ START	ASLEEP TIME	TOTAL TIME

_____'S SLEEP MANNERS CHART

	MONDAY	TUESDAY	WEDNESDAY	THURSDAY	FRIDAY	SATURDAY	SUNDAY
I LISTENED AND FOLLOWED DIRECTIONS AT BEDTIME							
I WENT TO SLEEP WITHOUT MOMMY LYING DOWN WITH ME							
I WENT BACK TO SLEEP ON MY OWN OVERNIGHT							
I STAYED IN BED UNTIL MY LIGHT CAME ON							

www.sleeplady.com

www.behavioristnextdoor.com

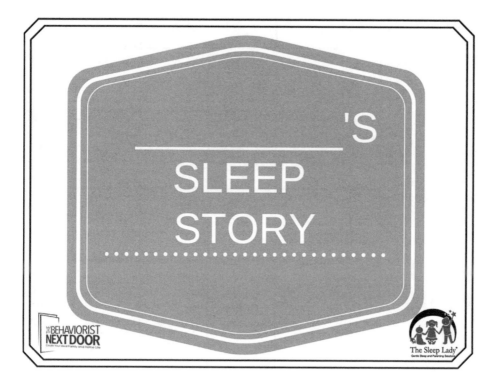

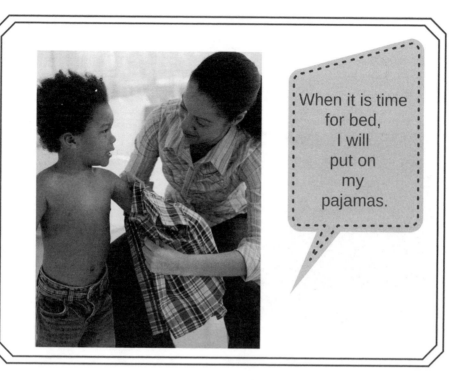

When it is time
for bed,
I will
put on
my
pajamas.

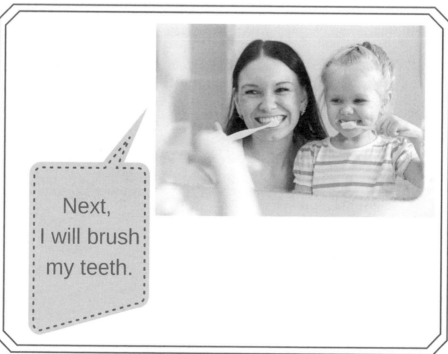

Next,
I will brush
my teeth.

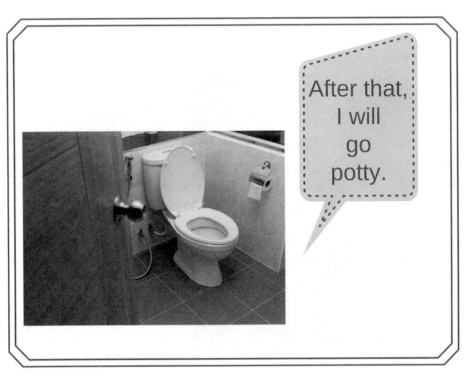

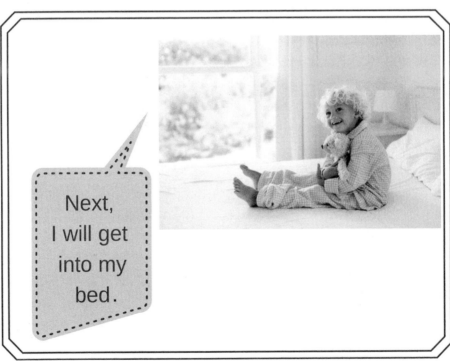

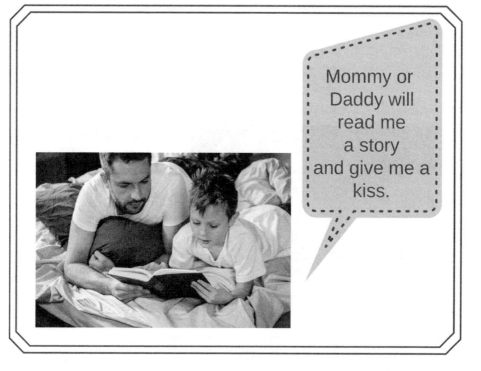

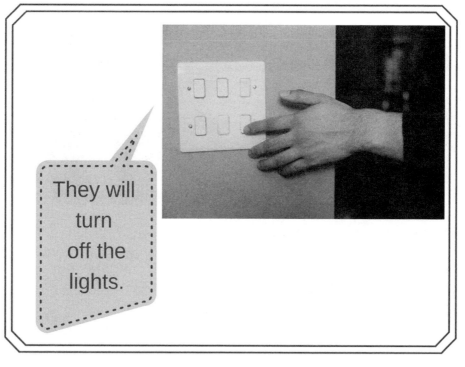

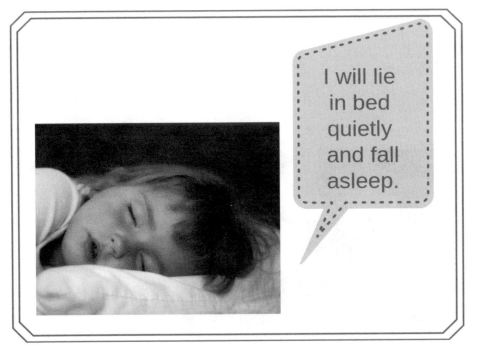

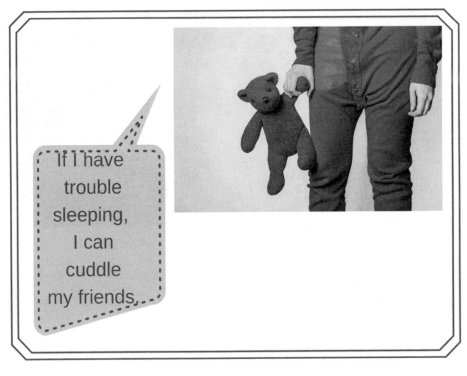

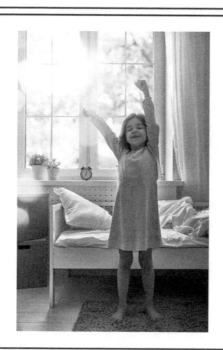

I feel great when I sleep in my bed all night!

I will get a sticker when I follow my sleep manners chart!

Bedtime Checklist

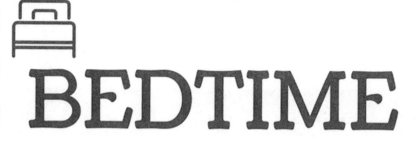

BEDTIME

PASS

This pass can be used for one more snuggle, kiss, or drink

www.sleeplady.com   www.behavioristnextdoor.com

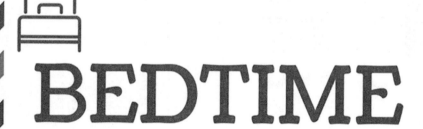

BEDTIME

PASS

This pass can be used for one more snuggle, kiss, or drink

www.sleeplady.com   www.behavioristnextdoor.com

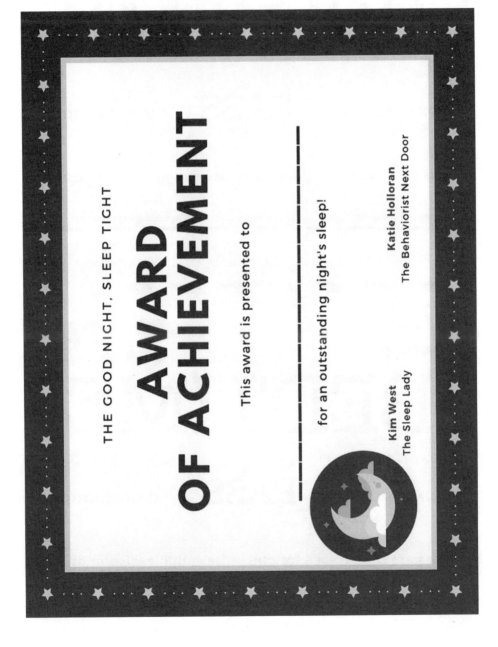

THE GOOD NIGHT, SLEEP TIGHT

AWARD
OF ACHIEVEMENT

This award is presented to

for an outstanding night's sleep!

Kim West
The Sleep Lady

Katie Holloran
The Behaviorist Next Door

CHAPTER FIFTEEN

Helpful Resources and Products For Sleep Training

Helpful Items for Your Home:

1. Sleep Sacks / Sheet Sets

2. Visual Clocks

3. Sound Machines

4. Vertical Crib Liners

5. Weighted Blankets

1. Sleep Sacks / Sheet Sets

Many families worry about their child's temperature at night, and wonder whether they are too cold. The general rule of thumb is for a child's room to be between 68 and 72 degrees Fahrenheit at night. Oftentimes, a child will push covers off while sleeping, causing him to wake up and need a parent to reorganize the sheets and blankets. Once a night or once in a while, this might be just fine, and not completely disruptive. However, if your child needs you to reset the sheets and blankets multiple times a night each and every night, it may help to find a toddler sleep sack or sheet set that can help alleviate this problem.

The Halo® SleepSack® Big Kids Wearable Blanket is a popular one with families. This wearable blanket provides comfort and warmth, along with a bit of mobility. **Find it at Buy Buy Baby, Amazon, Target**

Kids Zip Sheets® are an all-in-one sheet system. The top sheet zips up once the child is in bed, ensuring that they're snug in bed all night long, without needing to be re-tucked in multiple times. **Find it at www.kidszipsheets.com**

2. Visual Clocks

The Hatch Baby Rest is a visual clock and sound machine all in one. It can be programmed from your smartphone through a free app, and can be set to change colors at a set time so your child knows that when they see the color change, it's okay to get out of bed. **Find it at www.hatchbaby.com, Amazon, Target, or Bed, Bath & Beyond**

The OK to Wake! Alarm Clock & Night-Light is a helpful visual clock for children, especially when they cannot tell time yet. The clock has a setting that changes the color of the light when it is time to wake up. This way, your child will not be awakened by an alarm or sound; any time he wakes up, he will see whether it's "ok to wake" based on the color of the light. **Find it at Amazon, Target, or Bed, Bath & Beyond**.

Similar to the OK to Wake! clock, the Goodnitelite visual clock illuminates a blue moon during the night, and then a yellow sun when it is morning, at a time you set for your child. **Find it at www.goodnitelite.com, Amazon**

3. Sound Machine

Marpac® Dohm Elite White Noise Machine is a sound machine endorsed by the National Sleep Foundation as effectively masking disruptive noises to ensure a good night's sleep. This is a small machine that plugs into a standard outlet, and is easily portable, too. **Purchase at Amazon, Target, or Bed, Bath & Beyond**.

4. Vertical Crib Liners

While traditional crib bumpers are no longer recommended due to safety concerns, there are others on the market as of the writing of this workbook that help to keep kids' bodies safe while in the crib.

Pure Safety Vertical Crib Liners have been helpful for families with kids who bang their heads or bite on the crib while trying to soothe themselves to sleep. **Purchase at www.gomamagodesigns.com**

5. Weighted Blankets

Sleep researchers have noted that parents of children with special needs have reported increased sleep success (falling asleep faster, and waking up less at night) when children have slept with weighted blankets.

Talk with your child's pediatrician and/or occupational therapist about using them, and ask which one is recommended based on your child's needs. Your child's team likely has some favorites of their own.

Once you find one that is right for your child, use it just as you would a comforter or blanket on his bed. Tuck him in after your bedtime routine, and make sure he is snug and comfortable. Some kids notice the difference of the weight within seconds, and some don't notice any difference once under the blanket. While not all parents see marked results, some parents report that within a few days, the amount of time it takes a child to fall asleep has decreased measurably.

A few favorites from families we've known are listed here.

• Ball Blankets

One study showed that blankets filled with loose plastic balls helped children with AD/HD to fall asleep faster at bedtime. The balls in these blankets stimulate sensory receptors in the skin, muscles, and joints. **Find them at www.flaghouse.com/SensoryCritters-Ball-Blanket-item-34250**

- **Mosaic Weighted Blankets**

These blankets are quilted in squares with smaller pellets inside each square based on the particular weight you desire for your child. While this particular site has recommendations based on your child's weight, make sure to talk with your team about what would work best for your child. **Find them at www.mosaicweightedblankets.com**

Books

Siblings with Special Needs

Bourgeois, Paulette and Brenda Clark. *Franklin's Baby Sister*. Scholastic, 2000.

Brown, Marc. *Arthur's Baby*. Little, Brown, 1990.

DeMonia, Lori. *Leah's Voice*. Halo, 2012.

Elliott, Rebecca. *Just Because*. Lion Hudson, 2014.

Henkes, Kevin. *Julius, the Baby of the World*. HarperTrophy, 1995.

Lears, Laurie. *Ian's Walk: A Story About Autism*. Albert Whitman, 1998.

London, Jonathan. *Froggy's Baby Sister*. Viking, 2003.

Meyer, Mercer. *The New Baby*. Golden Books, 2001.

Peete, Holly Robinson and Peete, Ryan Elizabeth. *My Brother Charlie*. Scholastic, 2010.

Separation Anxiety/Anxious Kids

Heubner, Dawn. *What to Do When You Dread Your Bed: A Kid's Guide to Overcoming Problems with Sleep*. Magination Press, 2008.

_____. *What to Do When You Worry Too Much: A Kid's Guide to Overcoming Anxiety*. Magination Press, 2005.

Karst, Patrice. *The Invisible String*. Dvorss & Co, 2000.

Penn, Audrey. *The Kissing Hand*. Tanglewood Press, 2016.

Wright, Laurie. *I Can Handle It*. Laurie Wright, 2017.

Parent and Teacher Support Books

Barbera, Mary. *The Verbal Behavior Approach: How to Teach Children with Autism and Related Disorders*. Kingsley, 2007.

Cooper-Kahn. *Late, Lost, and Unprepared: A Parents' Guide to Helping Children with Executive Functioning*. Woodbine House, 2008.

Cooper-Kahn, Joyce and Foster, Margaret. *Boosting Executive Skills in the Classroom*. Jossey-Bass, 2013.

Dawson, Peg and Guare, Richard. *Smart But Scattered: The Revolutionary "Executive Skills" Approach to Helping Kids Reach Their Potential*. Guilford Press, 2009.

Gates, Miriam. *Good Night Yoga: A Pose-by-Pose Bedtime Story*. Sounds True, 2015.

Greene, Ross. *The Explosive Child*. Harper, 2014.

Kranowitz, Carol. *The Out of Sync Child: Recognizing and Coping with Sensory Processing Disorder*. TarcherPerigee, 2006.

Kurcinka, Mary Sheedy. *Raising Your Spirited Child, Third Edition: A Guide for Parents Whose Child Is More Intense, Sensitive, Perceptive, Persistent, and Energetic*. William Morrow, 2015.

Madrigal, Stephanie. *Superflex . . . A Superhero Social Thinking Curriculum*. Thinking Social, 2008.

Websites

American Academy of Pediatrics

www.AAP.org

The official site with advice and information about a multitude of pediatric topics. Resources, books, and videos are available on this site. www.healthychildren.org (from the AAP).

American Academy of Sleep Medicine (formerly the American Sleep Disorders Association)

www.aasmnet.org

The website of this membership group of doctors and other professionals contains links to sleep resources and research and also directs patients to accredited sleep disorder centers (not all of which treat children).

Autism Speaks

www.autismspeaks.org

Sleep toolkit for children and teenagers: https://www.autismspeaks.org/tool-kit/atnair-p-strategies-improve-sleep-children-autism

Consumer Product Safety Commission

www.cpsc.gov

List of product recalls and safety requirements for various products such as cribs.

First Candle Organization: Helping Babies Survive and Thrive

www.firstcandle.org

800-221-7437

National Sleep Foundation

www.sleepfoundation.org

This nonprofit group addresses numerous sleep issues for children and adults. The website includes the group's new childhood sleep guidelines.

Sources

American Academy of Pediatrics. "American Academy of Pediatrics Supports Childhood Sleep Guidelines." June 2016. Retrieved from: https://www.aap.org/en-us/about-the-aap/aap-pressroom/pages/American-Academy-of-Pediatrics-Supports-Childhood-Sleep-Guidelines.aspx.

Biel, Lindsey and Peske, Nancy. *Raising a Sensory Smart Child: The Definitive Handbook for Helping Your Child with Sensory Processing Issues*. Penguin Books, 2009.

Chitty, Antonia and Dawson, Victoria. *Sleep and Your Special Needs Child.* Robert Hale, 2014.

Dorfman, Kelly. *Cure Your Child with Food: The Hidden Connection Between Nutrition and Childhood Ailments*. Workman Publishing Company, revised edition, 2013.

Durand, V. Mark. *Sleep Better: A Guide to Improving Sleep for Children with Special Needs.* Brookes Publishing, 2014.

Friman PC, Hoff KE, Schnoes C, Freeman KA, Woods DW, Blum N. The bedtime pass: an approach to bedtime crying and leaving the room. Archives of *Pediatric and Adolescent Medicine*. 1999; 153: pp. 1027–1029.

Hvolby A, Bilenberg N. Use of Ball Blanket in attention-deficit/hyper-activity disorder sleeping problems. *Nordic Journal of Psychiatry*. 2019; 65:2: pp. 89–94,.doi:10.3109/08039488.2010.501868.

Jin CS, Hanley GP, and Beaulieu L. An individualized and comprehensive approach to treating sleep problems in young children. *Journal of Applied Behavior Analysis*. 2013; 46: 161–180. doi:10.1002/jaba.16

Katz, Terry and Malow, Beth. *Solving Sleep Problems in Children with Autism Spectrum Disorders: A Guide For Frazzled Families.* Woodbine House, 2014.

Kranowitz, Carol. *The Out of Sync Child Has Fun: Activities for Kids with Sensory Processing Disorder*. Rev. Ed. TarcherPerigee, 2006.

Kuhn, B. "The Excuse-Me Drill: A Behavioral Protocol to Promote Independent Sleep Initiation Skills and Reduce Bedtime Problems in Young Children." *Behavioral Treatments for Sleep Disorders*. Elsevier Inc., 2011. doi: 10.1016/B978-0-12-381522-4.00031-6

Kuypers, Leah. *The Zones of Regulation*. Think Social Publishing, 2011.

National Sleep Foundation. (2015, February). National Sleep Foundation Recommends new Sleep Times. National Sleep Foundation. February 2015.Retrieved from: https://sleepfoundation.org/press-release/national-sleep-foundation-recommends-new-sleep-times

O'Brien, et al. Sleep disturbances in children with attention deficit hyperactivity disorder. (2003). *Pediatric Research*. 2003;54: 2: pp. 237–243.

Perlis, Michael, et al. *Behavioral Treatments for Sleep Disorders: A Comprehensive Primer of Behavioral Sleep Medicine Interventions.* Elsevier, 2011.

Piazza CC, Fisher WW. Bedtime Fading in the Treatment of Pediatric Insomnia. *Journal of Behavior Therapy and Experimental Psychiatry*. 2991; 22 (1): pp. 53–56.

Quine, L. Severity of sleep problems in children with severe learning difficulties: description or correlates. *Journal of Community & Applied Social Psychology*. 1992; 2(4): pp. 247–268.